About Diabetes

➤ Diabetes is a disease where the body does not control the amount of glucose (sugar) in the blood.

➤ As glucose builds up in your blood over time, it can damage your body.

➤ Symptoms include feeling more thirsty, hungry or tired than normal, blurry vision, losing weight and needing to urinate more often.

➤ There is no cure for diabetes. But you can manage your diabetes through healthy eating, exercise and medicine as prescribed.

➤ With the support of your care team, you will learn how to manage your diabetes so you can lead a normal, healthy life.

What is diabetes?

When you don't have enough insulin, we say that you have insulin deficiency.

When the insulin your body is making does not work the way it should, we say that you have insulin resistance.

Diabetes is a disease that keeps your body from using the energy (calories) from the food you eat. This can happen if your body is not making enough of a hormone called **insulin**. It can also happen if the insulin your body makes does not work the way it should.

Insulin is made in the **pancreas**. It helps your body use the nutrients in the food that you eat. Without enough insulin, these nutrients are not absorbed normally into body cells.

One of these nutrients, called **carbohydrate**, changes to **glucose** (sugar) in the blood. Normally, insulin carries glucose from the bloodstream into the body's cells. When this does not happen, glucose can build up in your blood.

The cells in the pancreas that make insulin are called beta-cells.

If you have too much glucose in your blood, we say that you have high blood glucose (high blood sugar, or **hyperglycemia**). This can lead to damage in many parts of your body, including your eyes, kidneys, heart, blood vessels, nerves and skin. If not treated, the damage can be severe over time.

There is no cure for diabetes. Once you develop diabetes, you will have it for the rest of your life. The good news is that you can manage your diabetes with proper diet, exercise and medicine.

Taking Charge of Your Diabetes

Taking Charge of Your Diabetes

Fairview Health Services

Fairview Press, Minneapolis

Published by Fairview Press, 2450 Riverside Avenue, Minneapolis, MN 55454. Fairview Press is a division of Fairview Health Services, a community-focused health system affiliated with the University of Minnesota and providing a complete range of services, from the prevention of illness and injury to care for the most complex medical conditions. For a free current catalog of Fairview Press titles, please call toll-free 1-800-544-8207. Or visit our Web site at www.fairview.org.

First printing: January 2006

Library of Congress Cataloging-in-Publication Data
Taking charge of your diabetes / Fairview Health Services.
    p. cm.
  ISBN-13: 978-1-57749-167-5 (pbk. : alk. paper)
  ISBN-10: 1-57749-167-X (pbk.)
  1. Diabetes--Popular works. I. Fairview Health Services.
  RC660.4.T353 2007
  616.4'62--dc22
                 2006026147

Printed in the United States of America
11 10 09 08 07 06   1 2 3 4 5 6 7 8

Editors: Carol Brunzell, Sue Erickson, MaryAnn Loftus, Teresa Pearson

Contributors: Cynthia Bartoo, Teresa Benge, Amanda Brummel, Amy Dronen, Molly Ekstrand, Dee Jones, Mary Lavelle, Mardelle Madsen, Julie Miller, Nancy Olson, Delaine Reiman, Cheryl Rutt, Peg Salonek, Carol Schneider, Kelly Stenzel, Adele West

Customized editions of this publication (imprinted with your institution's name, contact information, etc.) are also available. Contact Fairview Press at 612-672-4774 for pricing.

The information in this book should not replace the advice of your doctor. Always follow your doctor's instructions. Before having any test or treatment, talk to your doctor to be sure you fully understand the risks and benefits involved.

SMARTworks 520383 – REV 09/06

Contents

How common is diabetes?

Over 20 million Americans have diabetes. Of these, six million don't even know they have it. Diabetes affects 1 in every 18 people in this country.

Are there different kinds of diabetes?

There are three basic kinds of diabetes: type 1, type 2 and gestational diabetes.

Type 1 diabetes

Type 1 diabetes occurs when the cells that make insulin are destroyed by the body's immune system. The body can no longer make insulin on its own.

About 5 to 10 percent of people with diabetes have type 1 diabetes.

This type of diabetes used to be called "juvenile-onset" diabetes because it is most common in people under age 30. It has also been called "insulin-dependent" diabetes because the people who have it must take insulin to manage it.

Type 2 diabetes

Type 2 diabetes occurs when the cells in the body do not use insulin normally. Over time, the body cannot make as much insulin as it needs. This is the most common kind of diabetes.

Type 2 diabetes used to be called "adult-onset" diabetes because it occurred mainly in adults. It is becoming more common among young people as Americans of all ages gain weight and exercise less. You are more likely to get type 2 diabetes if you:

- are overweight

- are inactive

- are over age 45

- have a family history of type 2 diabetes

- are African American, Latino, Native American, Asian American or Pacific Islander

About 90 to 95 percent of people with diabetes have type 2 diabetes.

- have given birth to a baby weighing over 9 pounds, or have had gestational diabetes during a pregnancy

- have high blood pressure (140/90 or higher)

- have an HDL cholesterol ("good" cholesterol) of 35 or lower, or triglyceride level of 250 or higher.

Some risk factors, such as being overweight or inactive, can be controlled. This is why managing type 2 diabetes always involves healthy eating and exercise. It is also important to control blood pressure and cholesterol. People with type 2 diabetes often take diabetes pills as well. In time, many people need to take insulin to help manage their blood glucose.

Gestational diabetes

Gestational diabetes occurs only in pregnant women. If not treated, it can cause problems for both the mother and the baby. Gestational diabetes usually goes away after the baby is born. But women who have had it are likely to have it again in future pregnancies. They are also more likely to have type 2 diabetes later in life.

If you have ever had gestational diabetes, you are more like to develop type 2 diabetes.

What is pre-diabetes?

Before people get type 2 diabetes, they almost always have **pre-diabetes.** Pre-diabetes is when your blood glucose level is higher than normal, but not high enough to be called diabetes. Damage to your body, especially the heart and blood vessels, may already be occurring during pre-diabetes. Risk factors include:

- waist size greater than 35 inches for women or greater than 40 inches for men

- inactive lifestyle

- high blood pressure

- HDL ("good") cholesterol under 45 for men and under 55 for women

- triglycerides greater than 250

- above-normal blood glucose

If you have pre-diabetes, you may delay or prevent diabetes if you start making healthy choices now.

- age greater than 45

- history of gestational diabetes or having given birth to a baby weighing more than 9 pounds

- family history of diabetes.

If you have pre-diabetes, it is important to start making healthy choices now. You can delay or prevent diabetes by losing weight, choosing healthy foods and doing physical activity for at least 30 minutes on five or more days of the week.

How do you diagnose diabetes?

There are different lab tests to measure how much glucose (sugar) is in your blood. One of the tests is called a **fasting plasma glucose test.** Before this test, you are asked not to eat or drink anything for 12 hours. Then, blood is drawn to test for glucose.

- If your blood glucose is less than 100, you do not have diabetes.

- If it is between 100 and 125, you have pre-diabetes.

- If your blood glucose is 126 or higher on two different days, you have diabetes.

Another test is called a **random,** or **casual, blood glucose test.** This test can be done at any time during the day, whether you have fasted or not. If your blood glucose is 200 or more *and* you have symptoms of diabetes, then you have diabetes. Symptoms of diabetes include feeling more thirsty or hungry than usual, losing weight and needing to urinate more often.

A third test to check for diabetes is the **oral glucose tolerance test.** For this test you must fast overnight (no eating or drinking). You will have a blood test, then you will drink a sweet liquid. Your blood will be tested again two more times: 1 hour and 2 hours later.

- If your blood glucose after two hours is less than 140, you do not have diabetes.

- If your blood glucose after two hours is between 140 and 199, you have pre-diabetes.

- If your blood glucose after two hours is greater than 200, you have diabetes.

Will I die from diabetes?

If you have just learned you have diabetes, your first reaction may be fear. You may wonder, What will diabetes do to my life? What will it do to my body? Am I going to die? How will my life change?

If you do not work to manage your diabetes, it can lead to serious problems, including death. But most problems can be avoided—if you're willing to make changes in your life.

If you learn about diabetes and take steps to control it, you will greatly reduce your risk of problems. But will life will go on as it did before you had diabetes? Yes and no.

You will have many of the same hobbies, routines and relationships as before, but you will need to make healthier choices. You will check your blood glucose often. You may need to take medicines. And you will actively work to prevent problems.

What should I do if I have diabetes?

Your first step is to learn how to manage your diabetes. Living well with diabetes means:

- eating healthy

- managing your weight

- being physically active

- managing your stress

- testing blood glucose often

- controlling blood pressure and cholesterol

- taking medicines as prescribed

It isn't easy to change your health habits, but your care team will help you every step of the way.

You will have to make some changes in your life. These changes may be among the hardest you'll ever make, but they're worth it. You can reduce your risk of long-term problems by managing your diabetes properly. You *can* take control of your life!

Chapter 2

Your Blood Glucose Levels

➤ "Blood glucose monitoring" means testing your blood glucose levels regularly.

➤ To test your blood glucose levels, you will do a simple blood test at home.

➤ This test is the only way to know if your blood glucose is high or low, and if your treatment plan is working.

➤ The test may sound scary at first, but it's quite easy to do.

➤ You will learn how to do this test, how often, and what glucose levels you should aim for.

What is blood glucose monitoring?

If you have diabetes or pre-diabetes, you should test the level of glucose in your blood. This involves testing a drop of your blood with a blood glucose meter.

How often you test your blood glucose will depend on your treatment plan. Please talk about your treatment plan with your diabetes care team.

Meeting your blood glucose goals will reduce your risk of health problems.

You will not be able to tell what your blood glucose level is based solely on how you feel. You must test your blood glucose with a meter. It is important to do this regularly, at home or wherever you are. This is the only way to know if your treatment plan is working and if you are meeting your blood glucose goals.

If you are not meeting your goals, you and your diabetes care team will need to make changes to your treatment plan.

Why should I test my blood glucose?

You should test your blood glucose:

- to know how your body is responding to food, exercise and medicine.

- to quickly tell if you have low blood glucose or high blood glucose.

- to know when to start or adjust your diabetes medicine.

- to know for sure what is happening with your blood glucose at any time.

- to keep your blood glucose levels in a normal range and lower your risk of health problems related to diabetes.

- because it's easy! You can take your blood glucose meter with you wherever you go.

Low blood glucose is called hypoglycemia. High blood glucose is called hyperglycemia.

How do I test my blood glucose?

1. Gather your equipment:

- **Blood glucose meter.** There are many different kinds of blood glucose meters. Work with your diabetes care team to choose the one that is best for you.

- **Test strip.** A test strip is a thin piece of special paper. You will place a drop of your blood on the paper for testing in your blood glucose meter. You will throw away the strip after you use it.

- **Lancet and lancing device.** A lancet is a sharp needle used to prick the finger to get a drop of blood. You will place the lancet into an automatic lancing device. This device "hides" the lancet and allows you to prick your finger without discomfort. After you use a lancet, you must throw it away in a safe container called a "sharps" container.

Diseases such as HIV and hepatitis can spread to others if they are pricked with a used lancet or needle that has infected blood on it.

- **Sharps container.** Lancets used for testing blood glucose and needles used for injecting insulin are called "sharps." Put these in a sharps container right after using them. Choose a container that:

  – you can close and seal tightly

  – will stand up straight and not tip over

  – will not leak, break, crack or let the sharps push through

- is clearly labeled

- is easy and safe to dispose of. (Most communities have rules for disposing sharps. Contact your garbage collection company for more information.)

- **Blood glucose record book or journal.** Keeping good records of your blood glucose levels will help you and your diabetes care team manage your diabetes better.

2. **Wash your hands in warm, soapy water.** Rinse and dry them completely.

3. **Prepare your finger for lancing.** First, hang your hand at your side for a few seconds. Shake your hand as if you were trying to flip water off it. Then, squeeze your finger above the middle knuckle while holding it below heart level.

4. **Set up your meter.** Use your meter as instructed by the manufacturer. If you have questions, call the toll-free number on the back of the meter for help.

5. **Lance (prick) your finger.** Use your lancing device to prick your finger, then squeeze out a drop of blood. Prick the side of your finger, not the pad of your finger. (If you wish, you may ask your care team about using another part of your body.)

Prick the side of your finger, not the pad of your finger.

6. **Put the blood on the test strip.** Follow the instructions that came with your meter. Read your results.

7. **Write your results in your record book.** If your blood glucose level is above or below your target range, take a moment to think about why this might be. Write a short note about it in your record book.

8. **Remove the lancet from the lancing device.** Throw the lancet away in your sharps container. You may throw the test strip in the garbage.

When should I test my blood glucose?

Ask your diabetes care team when and how often you should test your blood glucose. Here are some suggested times:

Before breakfast. This will tell you what your blood glucose is after 8 to 10 hours of fasting.

Before meals. This will tell you what your blood glucose level is when you have not eaten for a few hours.

After meals. Testing two hours after you start eating will tell you how the food you ate affects your blood glucose.

Testing your blood glucose is the only way to know if your glucose is too low or too high.

Before bed. Before you go to sleep, your blood glucose needs to be at a safe level. Discuss your bedtime target range with your care team.

Before and after physical activities. Testing before exercise helps you see if you need a snack before you begin. Testing after exercise helps you see how the activity affected your blood glucose.

When you have symptoms of hypoglycemia (low blood glucose). This lets you be sure that your blood glucose really is low before you try to do anything about it. If you are unable to test your blood glucose, or you do not have your meter with you, eat or drink something that contains carbohydrate (see chapter 4).

Blood glucose can rise when you are sick.

When you are sick. The level of glucose in your blood can rise when you are sick, so you may need to test your blood glucose more often than usual. Work with your diabetes care team to plan for those days when you feel sick.

What should my glucose level be?

Taking good care of your diabetes involves testing your blood glucose levels every day. This way, you will always know what your blood glucose is, and you will know right away if you may need to change your meal plan, exercise plan or medicine. Ask your diabetes care team when and how often you should test your blood glucose.

Blood Glucose Goals for People with Diabetes

When you check blood glucose . . .	Your level should be . . .
Before meals	90 to 130
2 hours after meals	Less than 180
At bedtime	100 to 140
Your A1c should be less than 7%	

What Is a Hemoglobin A1c Test?

A hemoglobin A1c test is a blood test. It averages the amount of glucose in the blood over three months. Studies have shown that people with diabetes can lower their risk of complications if the average amount of glucose in their blood over three months is less than 7%.

People without diabetes have an A1c range of 4 to 6%. If your A1c is 7% or higher, you should review your treatment plan with your diabetes care team.

My A1c is _____.

Most people should schedule an A1c test every 3 to 6 months. Remember:

If your A1c level is . . .	Your average glucose level is . . .
4%	65
5%	100
6%	135
7%	170
8%	205
9%	240
10%	275
11%	310
12%	345
13%	380

When should I call my doctor?

Call your doctor when:

- Your blood glucose is **often** over your goal.

- Your blood glucose is **often** low (hypoglycemia).

- You are sick, and your sick-day plan says you should call your doctor.

- You have questions or concerns about your diabetes treatment plan or your medicines.

Make sure to have the following information ready to give your doctor:

- your blood glucose numbers

- the times of the day you took your diabetes medicine

- the amount and type of diabetes medicine you took

- your temperature, if you are sick

- any other medicines or recent changes in your lifestyle.

Chapter 3

Know Your Diabetes Medicines

➤ Medicine can be used to keep blood glucose (sugar) levels as close to normal as possible. Most people need medicine to help manage their diabetes.

➤ All people who have type 1 diabetes must take insulin. People who have type 2 diabetes may take diabetes pills, insulin or other medicine.

➤ Some people can manage their diabetes through diet and exercise and may not need medicine.

➤ It's important to know how much medicine to take, when to take it and what side effects to watch for.

➤ If you have any questions about your medicine, call your doctor or care team. They are here to help you.

Insulin is a hormone made in the pancreas. It helps keep your blood glucose levels normal by moving glucose from your bloodstream into your cells, where it is used for energy.

There are two main forms of diabetes medicine: pills and shots. Shots may contain insulin or another type of medicine.

All people with type 1 diabetes need to take insulin. Some people with type 2 diabetes can control their diabetes with diet and exercise alone. But when these are not enough, they need to take diabetes medicine.

Many people believe that diabetes pills are insulin. They are not. In fact, your body must be making its own insulin for some diabetes pills to work.

No matter what type of diabetes medicine you take, your goal will always be the same: to keep the level of glucose in your blood as close to normal as possible.

Safe Medicines

Before you begin taking any medicine, you should know the answers to the following questions.

- What medicine will I be taking?
- What is it for?

- How much will I take, and when?
- What are the side effects?

- What do I do if I forget to take it?
- Should I still take it if I get sick?

Diabetes pills (oral medicines)

Biguanides

Example: Metformin (Glucophage)

How it works: Causes the liver to release less glucose and helps muscle cells use insulin. May help you lose weight. Lowers the levels of fats and cholesterol in your blood.

Side effects:

- Nausea, diarrhea, loss of appetite. These side effects should go away within a few weeks. To reduce them, take the medicine with food or milk.

- Lactic acidosis is a rare but serious side effect. This can occur in people who have kidney or severe lung problems.

Warnings: Metformin may not be right for you if you:

- have kidney or severe lung problems.

- are 80 years of age or older.

- are taking medicine for heart failure.

- have a history of liver disease or alcohol abuse.

One advantage of using metformin is it will not cause you to gain weight.

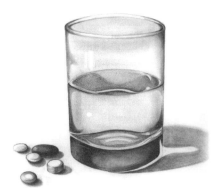

If you are scheduled for any test or procedure where you will have an iodine dye injected into your veins, tell your doctor that you take metformin. You should not take it for at least 2 days after the test or procedure.

Thiazolidinediones

Examples: Rosiglitazone (Avandia), pioglitazone (Actos)

How it works: Helps your muscle cells use insulin. Usually takes 4 to 6 weeks to lower blood glucose.

Side effects:

You may need regular blood tests if you take certain diabetes medicines.

- Can cause you to gain weight, so it is important to eat wisely and exercise regularly while taking this medicine.

- Can affect your liver. You should have a blood test to check your liver before starting this medicine. Your doctor will test your liver regularly while you are taking it. Call your doctor at once if you have any signs of liver damage, including:

  - feeling sick to your stomach

  - throwing up

  - pain in your abdomen (belly)

  - feeling very tired

  - not feeling hungry

  - dark urine.

- Can cause fluid build-up or swelling.

- Can cause women who are not ovulating (and who have not gone through menopause) to begin ovulating again. This would make it possible for a woman to get pregnant.

Warnings:

- You should not take this medicine if you have heart failure.

- Women who are not ovulating may need birth control to prevent pregnancy.

- Birth control pills may not work as well with this medicine. Women should discuss other options with their doctor.

Birth control pills may not work well with this medicine. Use another form of birth control, even if you think you can't get pregnant.

Sulfonylureas

Examples: Glimepiride (Amaryl), glipizide (Glucotrol), glyburide (Diabeta, Micronase, Glynase PresTab)

How it works: Helps the pancreas release more insulin. Similar to meglitinides, but works for a longer period of time. Can raise insulin levels for several hours.

Side effects: Can cause hypoglycemia (low blood glucose), especially if you take too much, delay or skip a meal, do more exercise than normal or drink alcohol on an empty stomach.

Meglitinides

Examples: Repaglinide (Prandin), nateglinide (Starlix)

How it works: Helps the pancreas release more insulin. Similar to sulfonylureas, but works for a shorter length of time.

Side effects: Can cause hypoglycemia (low blood glucose), especially if you delay or skip a meal, exercise more than normal, drink alcohol on an empty stomach or take too much of this medicine. This is less likely than if you take sulfonylureas.

Warnings:

- Don't take this medicine if you are skipping a meal or you are having hypoglycemia.

- Ask your doctor if you should take it before eating large snacks.

Alpha-glucosidase inhibitors

Examples: Acarbose (Precose), miglitol (Glyset)

How it works: Helps the intestines digest and absorb carbohydrates more slowly. This keeps blood glucose from rising too high after a meal.

Side effects:

- Gas, bloating, diarrhea. To reduce these side effects, your doctor may have you start with a low dose and increase the dose slowly.

- May cause hypoglycemia (low blood glucose) when used with a sulfonylurea or insulin. Treat hypoglycemia with glucose tablets or gels. (Eating carbohydrates will not work as fast because the medicine slows the breakdown of carbohydrates.)

Warnings: People with inflammatory bowel disease (IBD) and other intestinal diseases or obstructions should not take this medicine.

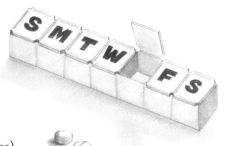

Combination medicines

Examples:

- Metformin and glyburide (Glucovance)

- Metformin and rosiglitazone (Avandamet)

- Metformin and glipizide (Metaglip)

- Rosiglitazone and glimepiride (Avandaryl)

- Rosiglitazone and metformin (Actoplus Met)

Diabetes shots (injectable medicines)

Exenatide (Byetta)

How it works:

- Helps the pancreas make the right amount of insulin at the right time.

- Slows the rate at which glucose enters your bloodstream, preventing spikes in glucose.

- Reduces the amount of glucose released from the liver when you don't need it.

- Decreases appetite, which may result in weight loss.

Side effects: Can cause weight loss and nausea. Nausea usually improves with time. May also cause hypoglycemia (low blood glucose) when used with a sulfonylurea.

Warnings:

- Do not take this medicine if you have severe kidney disease, gastroparesis or severe gastrointestinal disease.

- If you take a sulfonylurea, you will need to reduce your sulfonylurea dose when starting this medicine.

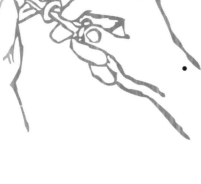

Pramlintide (Symlin)

How it works: Lowers blood glucose right after a meal by slowing the rate at which food empties from your stomach. May also reduce the amount of glucose released from the liver after a meal. Decreases appetite so you will eat less.

Side effects: Can cause nausea, vomiting, weight loss and low blood glucose.

Warnings:

- You should not take this medicine if:
    - Your A1c is over 9%.
    - You often have low blood glucose.
    - You have gastroparesis.
    - You take any medicine that affects the rate at which the stomach empties.

- This medicine is used in people who take insulin at mealtime. To avoid hypoglycemia, you will need to reduce your insulin by half when starting this medicine.

Insulin

Many people with type 2 diabetes eventually need to take insulin to manage their blood glucose. This is because the cells that make insulin wear out over time. The longer you have diabetes, the less likely it is that your cells will make enough insulin.

Insulin does a very good job of lowering blood glucose. Taking insulin does not mean that your diabetes is "getting worse." It just means that you are using another tool to help you manage your blood glucose.

How does it work?

Insulin lowers blood glucose by moving glucose from the bloodstream into the cells of the body, where it is used for energy.

There are four main types of insulin:

- Rapid-acting insulin such as lispro (Humalog), aspart (Novolog) or glulisine (Apidra)

- Short-acting insulin (regular)

- Intermediate-acting insulin (NPH)

- Long-acting insulin such as glargine (Lantus) or detemir (Levemir).

Type of insulin	How fast it works	When it peaks	How long it works
Rapid-acting • *lispro (Humalog);* • *aspart (Novolog);* • *glulisine (Apidra)*	15 minutes *(for all)*	30 minutes to 1½ hours *(for all)*	3 to 5 hours *(for all)*
Short-acting • *regular*	30 minutes to 1 hour	2 to 3 hours	6 to 8 hours
Intermediate-acting • *NPH*	1 hour to 1½ hours	6 to 8 hours	12 to 18 hours
Long-acting • *glargine (Lantus)* • *detemir (Levemir)*	*glargine:* 2 hours *detemir:* 3 to 4 hours	*glargine:* no peak *detemir:* minimal peak 6 to 8 hours	*glargine:* 24 hours *detemir:* up to 24 hours

How do I take it?

Most insulin is given as a shot through a syringe or insulin pen. Your care team will show you how to give yourself a shot. A new type of insulin can be inhaled. Your doctor can tell you if inhaled insulin is right for you.

Insulin does not come in pill form. If you took insulin as a pill, your body would digest it and it would be destroyed.

How much do I take?

The dose and type of insulin will vary from person to person, and it will change according to your blood glucose results. Your care team will tell you how much to take and when to take it.

What are the side effects?

Insulin can cause hypoglycemia (low blood glucose). If you need insulin to help lower your blood glucose, talk with your diabetes care team about how to avoid hypoglycemia.

What is Exubera (inhaled insulin)?

Exubera is a rapid-acting insulin to be inhaled less than 10 minutes before eating. For type 1 diabetes, you still need long-acting insulin shots if you use Exubera. For type 2 diabetes, you can use it with or without diabetes pills or long-acting insulin.

Exubera may cause low blood glucose, dry mouth, chest pain and cough. For most people, the chest pain and cough are mild and temporary. Tell your care team if symptoms are severe or if they persist.

Some people who take inhaled insulin must continue taking insulin shots as well.

Do not use this medicine if you smoke, have quit smoking within the past six months, or have lung disease (including asthma, emphysema and chronic obstructive pulmonary disease). You should have your lungs tested before starting this medicine, six months after using it, and then yearly after that.

Wear Your Medical ID

If you faint or cannot speak for yourself, medical identification (ID) will tell care providers how to treat you.

You should wear medical ID if you take insulin or other diabetes medicine. The ID should list any medical problems you have, including diabetes.

You can buy the ID from most drug stores, jewelry stores and companies that advertise in diabetes magazines. Ask your care team which ID will work best for you:

- Wrist or ankle bracelet

- Necklace

- Neck chain with military-style tags

- Watch charms

- Shoe tags

It's a good idea to carry a wallet card with your medical information as well.

What about over-the-counter medicine?

Some nonprescription drugs may affect your blood glucose. For information about over-the-counter medicines, see chapter 8, "Day-to-Day Living."

Chapter 4

Hypoglycemia and Hyperglycemia

➤ HypOglycemia is low blood glucose (low blood sugar). HypERglycemia is high blood glucose.

➤ Your risk for hypoglycemia is very low unless you take certain medicines (sulfonylureas, meglitinides or insulin).

➤ Blood glucose levels change with food, exercise, medicine, stress and illness.

➤ You can help prevent problems by eating the right amount of food at the right time, taking medicines as prescribed, getting regular exercise and testing your blood glucose often.

What is hypoglycemia?

Hypoglycemia is low blood glucose (sugar). It is sometimes called "insulin reaction" or "insulin shock." When your blood glucose level goes below 70 or you have certain symptoms, we say that you have hypoglycemia.

Usually, hypoglycemia is mild and easy to treat. But if it is not treated quickly, it can be serious.

Why would my blood glucose be low?

Your blood glucose may be low if you are:

People who take insulin, sulfonylureas or meglitinides may sometimes get hypoglycemia.

- skipping or not finishing meals or snacks.

- taking too high a dose of certain medicines (sulfonylureas, meglitinides or insulin).

- eating meals or snacks at the wrong time.

- exercising more than usual or harder than usual.

- drinking too much alcohol or drinking on an empty stomach.

- under stress.

- taking medicines or herbs that affect your blood glucose.

How do I know if I have low blood glucose?

You may have hypoglycemia if:

- your heart begins to beat fast

- your lips or mouth feel numb or tingly

- you feel shaky

- you start sweating

- you feel nervous, crabby or confused

- you have a headache

- you cannot see well

- you feel dizzy, tired or weak

- you are suddenly very hungry.

Symptoms tend to happen in the same order over and over. Try to learn what your first symptoms are so you can treat low blood glucose right away.

If possible, test your blood glucose. This is the only way to know for sure if you have hypoglycemia.

Sometimes symptoms will occur at night. If you are restless, sweating, having nightmares or waking up with headaches, you may have low blood glucose. To find out, your care team may ask you to test your blood glucose in the middle of your sleep period.

How should I treat low blood glucose?

Low blood glucose will not get better on its own. You will need to treat it as soon as possible.

You need to treat hypoglycemia as soon as possible. It will not get better on its own.

1. **Test your blood glucose.**

2. **Eat or drink carbohydrate right away.**

    *   **If your blood glucose is less than 70,** or if you have any symptoms of low blood glucose, eat or drink something with 15 grams of carbohydrate. The following have about 15 grams of carbohydrate:

        - 3 to 4 glucose tablets

        - ½ cup of regular soda pop (soda pop with sugar, not diet soda pop)

        - ½ cup fruit juice

        - 1 small box of raisins

        - 6 or 7 hard candies (not sugar-free; chewed, not sucked)

        - 1 cup of skim milk

        - 1 tablespoon of honey or sugar

        - 5 small sugar cubes

    *   **If your glucose is less than 50 the first time you check it,** eat a double serving from this list (about 30 grams of carbohydrate).

3. **Wait at least 5 minutes before eating anything else.** Most people feel much better in 5 to 10 minutes. Try not to eat more carbohydrate until you retest your blood glucose.

If you think you have low blood glucose but cannot test your blood, eat or drink one of the items listed here.

4. **Retest your blood glucose in 10 to 15 minutes.** If it is still less than 70, eat or drink another 15 grams of carbohydrate.

Keep checking your blood glucose every 15 minutes. Repeat the steps above if needed.

If your next meal is more than an hour away, eat another 15 to 30 grams of carbohydrate. This is even more important if you are doing physical activity such as housework, yard work, shopping or exercise. Test your blood glucose again in one hour.

If you are unable to treat yourself: Someone else can give you the carbohydrate you need. If you cannot swallow, they can give you a shot of glucagon (medicine to treat low blood glucose). Ask your care team of glucagon is right for you.

Call your doctor or dial 911 if your blood glucose does not get better.

Glucagon Kit

This contains emergency medicine (glucagon) for treating severe low blood glucose when you are unable to treat yourself. It will be important for those around you to know how to use the kit.

Keep the kit with you at all times. If you faint from low blood glucose, the people who are with you can give you the medicine you need.

Rebound Hyperglycemia

After you treat hypoglycemia, your glucose may rise too high as your body tries to adjust. This is called "rebound hyperglycemia." It can last for up to 24 hours. Blood glucose can also get too high if you eat too much carbohydrate to treat your hypoglycemia.

Try to follow the steps listed here to treat low blood glucose. This may help prevent problems later.

If you know why your blood glucose was low, you can take steps to keep it from happening again.

How do I prevent low blood glucose?

Whenever you have low blood glucose, it is important to try to understand how it may have happened. This way you can reduce the risk of it happening again.

Think back to a few hours before you had hypoglycemia. What did you do—or not do—that may have caused your blood glucose to be low?

You can prevent low blood glucose by:

- eating the right amount of food at the right time

- always eating a meal or snack that contains carbohydrate when drinking alcohol

- taking the right amount of diabetes medicine at the right time

- getting regular exercise

- exercising one hour after a meal, not before a meal

- checking and recording your blood glucose levels regularly.

Keep talking to your diabetes care team. They may need to change your treatment plan to help you manage your blood glucose.

Let your diabetes care team know if:

- you have more than two to three low blood glucose readings in a row.

- you have two or more low readings in 24 hours.

- you have low readings at the same time of day several days in a row.

- you need to eat extra food to keep your blood glucose from falling.

If one or more of these things is happening to you, your treatment plan may need to change. You may need to take less medicine or change to a different medicine.

Safety Tips

Tell family, friends, exercise partners, coworkers and classmates that you have diabetes. Let them know how they can help you if you have low blood glucose.

Always carry some form of carbohydrate with you.

Always test your blood glucose before you drive. You should never drive when your blood glucose is low. If you think you are low, pull off the road and treat the low blood glucose.

Always wear or carry identification (ID) that says you have diabetes. If you can't talk, this will let people know what's wrong and get you the care you need.

If you have hypoglycemia, try to remember the first symptom that told you something was wrong. If you know the first feeling you have of low blood glucose, you can treat it before it gets worse.

You can get hypoglycemia even when you and your diabetes care team are working hard to control your diabetes. It does not mean that you or anyone else has done something wrong.

What is hyperglycemia?

Hyperglycemia means having blood glucose levels that are higher than your goal.

What are the symptoms of high blood glucose?

Symptoms may include feeling more thirsty, tired or hungry than normal; blurry vision; losing weight and needing to urinate more often.

Call your doctor if your blood glucose is often over 180. This means you have hyperglycemia. Your doctor may need to adjust your treatment plan.

What makes my blood glucose high?

There are many reasons why your blood glucose may be high:

- You may be eating too much.

- You may have an illness or infection.

- You may not be getting the right amount or the right type of diabetes medicine.

- You may be stressed.

- Your hormones may be affecting you.

- You may not be getting enough physical activity.

- You may be taking medicines that can raise your blood glucose.

What should I do if I think I have high blood glucose?

You may be able to lower your blood glucose level by exercising more and eating less. If exercise and diet changes don't help, your doctor may change your medicines.

Without treatment, high blood glucose can lead to **ketoacidosis.** This occurs in a small number of people. Symptoms include:

- vomiting (throwing up)

- weakness

- rapid breathing

- sweet-smelling breath.

This is a serious problem. If you have any of these symptoms, call your doctor at once.

Know when to call for help! If you have these symptoms, you may need treatment right away.

How do I prevent high blood glucose?

Everyone who has diabetes will have high blood glucose at times. You can help prevent it by:

- eating the right amount of food at the right time

- taking the right amount of diabetes medicine at the right time

- getting regular exercise

- checking and recording your blood glucose levels regularly.

Call your doctor if your blood glucose level is often above your goal.

Hyperglycemia
(high blood glucose)

Happens slowly. May lead to serious illness, including coma.

Symptoms:
- Extreme thirst
- Urinating more often
- Dry skin
- Hunger
- Blurred vision
- Feeling drowsy
- Slow healing after illness or injury

Causes:
- Too much food
- Wrong type or amount of diabetes medicine
- Stress or illness
- Lack of exercise

What to do:
- Exercise more and eat less.
- Test your blood glucose regularly.
- Call your doctor if your glucose level is often above your goal.

Symptoms:
- Shaking, sweating, fast heartbeat
- Feeling dizzy, tired and weak
- Feeling anxious and irritable
- Hunger
- Vision problems, headache
- Numb or tingling mouth

Causes:
- Too little food, or eating at the wrong times
- Too much diabetes medicine
- More activity than normal
- Stress, alcohol, some medicines

What to do:
- Test your blood glucose.
  - If under 70: have ½ cup juice or 1 Tbsp sugar.
  - If under 50: have 1 cup juice or 2 Tbsp sugar.
- Repeat every 15 minutes until glucose is normal.
- Call your doctor or 911 if glucose does not improve.

Happens fast.
May lead to insulin shock.

(low blood glucose)
Hypoglycemia

Chapter 5

Healthy Eating

➤ A healthy diet is one of the most important parts of managing diabetes.

➤ You can start by eating more fresh fruits, vegetables and whole grains.

➤ Changing your diet doesn't have to be hard. As you try new foods and make healthy choices, your tastes will change. In time, many people say they like the healthy foods better!

Choosing healthy foods is always an important part of living well with diabetes. Besides making you healthier overall, healthy eating will help you to control your blood glucose, cholesterol, blood pressure and weight.

There is no "special" diet for people with diabetes. The foods recommended for good health are the same for all people, whether they have diabetes or not.

- **Eat many different kinds of foods** from the basic food groups.

- **Control the number of calories you eat and drink** to help you manage your weight.

- **Choose your carbohydrates wisely.** For example, eat more fruits and vegetables and whole grains rather than processed and refined foods.

- **Limit the amount of fat you eat.** When you do eat fat, try to choose fats that come from plants rather than animals. Choose monounsaturated fats or polyunsaturated fats (like the fats in olive oil, canola oil or nuts). Limit saturated fats or trans fats (like the fats in butter, lard or hydrogenated oils).

- **Reduce the amount of sodium (salt) that you eat.**

Try to replace white bread with whole wheat bread. Replace white rice with brown rice.

Avoid any foods that list the words "hydrogenated" or "partially hydrogenated" on the label. These contain trans fats.

- **If you drink alcohol, do so in moderation.**

- **Keep foods safe to eat.**
  - Keep hot foods hot, and cold foods cold.
  - Note the expiration dates on packages. (These are sometimes called "best before" dates or "use by" dates.)
  - Wash fruits and vegetables well.
  - Do not let raw meat touch other foods. Wash anything that touches raw meat with hot, soapy water.
  - Wash your hands often when handling and making food.

To find out how many calories and food servings are right for you, talk to your diabetes educator. Or go to MyPyramid.gov.

The guidelines on the next page gives a basic introduction to good nutrition.

GRAINS
Make half your grains whole

Eat at least 3 oz. of whole-grain cereals, breads, crackers, rice, or pasta every day

1 oz. is about 1 slice of bread, about 1 cup of breakfast cereal, or ½ cup of cooked rice, cereal, or pasta

VEGETABLES
Vary your veggies

Eat more dark-green veggies like broccoli, spinach, and other dark leafy greens

Eat more orange vegetables like carrots and sweetpotatoes

Eat more dry beans and peas like pinto beans, kidney beans, and lentils

FRUITS
Focus on fruits

Eat a variety of fruit

Choose fresh, frozen, canned, or dried fruit

Go easy on fruit juices

MILK
Get your calcium-rich foods

Go low-fat or fat-free when you choose milk, yogurt, and other milk products

If you don't or can't consume milk, choose lactose-free products or other calcium sources such as fortified foods and beverages

MEAT & BEANS
Go lean with protein

Choose low-fat or lean meats and poultry

Bake it, broil it, or grill it

Vary your protein routine — choose more fish, beans, peas, nuts, and seeds

---

For a 2,000-calorie diet, you need the amounts below from each food group. To find the amounts that are right for you, go to MyPyramid.gov.

Eat 6 oz. every day | **Eat 2½ cups every day** | **Eat 2 cups every day** | **Get 3 cups every day;** for kids aged 2 to 8, it's 2 | **Eat 5½ oz. every day**

Find your balance between food and physical activity

- Be sure to stay within your daily calorie needs.
- Be physically active for at least 30 minutes most days of the week.
- About 60 minutes a day of physical activity may be needed to prevent weight gain.
- For sustaining weight loss, at least 60 to 90 minutes a day of physical activity may be required.
- Children and teenagers should be physically active for 60 minutes every day, or most days.

Know the limits on fats, sugars, and salt (sodium)

- Make most of your fat sources from fish, nuts, and vegetable oils.
- Limit solid fats like butter, stick margarine, shortening, and lard, as well as foods that contain these.
- Check the Nutrition Facts label to keep saturated fats, *trans* fats, and sodium low.
- Choose food and beverages low in added sugars. Added sugars contribute calories with few, if any, nutrients.

MyPyramid.gov
STEPS TO A HEALTHIER YOU

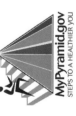

U.S. Department of Agriculture
Center for Nutrition Policy and Promotion
April 2005
CNPP-15

USDA is an equal opportunity provider and employer.

Calories

A calorie is a measure of the amount of energy in food. Calories are found in almost all foods. They come from carbohydrates, protein, fat and alcohol.

What do calories have to do with body weight?

If you burn off more energy, or calories, than you eat, you will lose weight. If you burn the same number of calories as you eat, your weight will stay the same. If you burn fewer calories than you eat, you will gain weight.

A gram of carbohydrate and a gram of protein each has 4 calories. A gram of fat has 9 calories. A gram of alcohol has 7 calories.

What does body weight have to do with diabetes?

For many people with type 2 diabetes, losing just 5 to 10 percent of their body weight—or about 10 to 20 pounds—would improve their blood glucose, cholesterol and blood pressure. To see what a healthy body weight would be for you, go to the Body Mass Index at the end of this chapter.

How can I lose weight?

The best way to lose weight is by controlling how much you eat (eat fewer calories), what you eat (eat healthy foods), and how much energy you use (burn more calories).

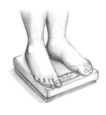

Nutrients

Nutrients are the things in the foods you eat that your body needs to be healthy. There are six different nutrients in foods:

- carbohydrates

- proteins

- fats

- vitamins

- minerals

- water.

Carbohydrates

Carbohydrates are your body's main source of energy. There are three basic types: starches, sugars and fiber.

Try to eat the same amount of carbohydrate foods at the same times each day.

The body breaks down starches and sugars into glucose. (Fiber does not affect blood glucose.) Insulin then carries this glucose through the bloodstream to the cells of the body. The cells use the glucose for energy.

Because carbohydrates contain the vitamins and minerals you need for good health, they are an important part of a healthy diet.

Will some carbohydrates affect my blood glucose more than others?

All foods with starches and sugars will affect your blood glucose in about the same way when eaten in equal amounts. Eating about the same amounts of carbohydrate at about the same times each day will help keep your blood glucose in your target range.

Your dietitian will show you how much carbohydrate you should eat for each meal and snack.

What Foods Contain Carbohydrates?

Starches and sugars are found in:

- grains and grain products, including breads, cereals, pasta and rice

- starchy vegetables, including corn, peas, potatoes and winter squash

- dried peas, beans and other legumes

- fresh, canned and dried fruits and fruit juices

- milk and yogurt

- desserts, snack foods and sweetened drinks.

What about fiber?

Fiber does not affect blood glucose, but eating fiber has been shown to help lower cholesterol. It also helps to prevent constipation (hard stools).

Next time you shop for groceries, look for whole wheat pasta instead of white pasta.

Fiber is found in:

- whole grains

- whole fruits and vegetables

- dried peas, beans and other legumes

- nuts and seeds.

There are two types of fiber in foods.

Add fiber to your diet slowly. For example, you can mix brown and white rice, using less white rice over time.

- **Soluble fiber** helps to lower cholesterol. You can find soluble fiber in whole grain products made from oats, oat bran, brown rice, pumpernickel, rye, barley and soy; dried peas, beans and other legumes; and fresh fruits and vegetables.

- **Insoluble fiber** helps to prevent and treat constipation (hard stools). You can find insoluble fiber in whole wheat and bran products such as cereal, pasta, bread and crackers.

How much fiber should I eat?

Try to eat at least 20 to 35 grams of fiber per day. If you are not eating much fiber now, add it to your diet slowly to avoid gas, bloating or discomfort.

How can I add fiber to my diet?

Begin by replacing low-fiber foods with high-fiber foods.

- Eat whole grain bread rather than white bread. (Be careful. Many breads labeled "wheat" or "multigrain" bread are made with refined flours. Look for labels that say "whole wheat" or "whole grain" bread, or that list whole grains as the first ingredient.)

- Eat a baked potato with the skin on rather than mashed potatoes.

- Eat an apple with the skin instead of applesauce.

- Have fresh fruit instead of fruit juice.

- Eat popcorn rather than potato chips.

- Eat bran cereal rather than corn flakes.

- Add beans, peas and lentils to soups and stews.

Try eating fruits and vegetables with their skins on. Choose whole fruits rather than fruit juices.

For the fiber content of common foods, see the fiber table at the end of this chapter.

Protein

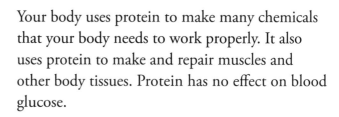

Your body uses protein to make many chemicals that your body needs to work properly. It also uses protein to make and repair muscles and other body tissues. Protein has no effect on blood glucose.

Protein is found in:

Instead of meat, try adding cooked beans or lentils to soups and stews. This way you get protein without the cholesterol.

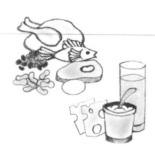

- beef, pork, lamb, veal and other meat products

- chicken, turkey and other poultry

- fish and other seafood

- eggs

- milk, cheese and yogurt

- dried peas and beans

- tofu and soy products

- nuts and nut butters.

Fats

Your body uses fat to help make cells, hormones and other chemicals that it needs to work properly. Fat is a good source of vitamins A, D, E and K.

While our bodies need some fat for good health, it is important to choose the right kinds of fat in the right amounts.

Try to use more vegetable fats (nuts, seeds, olive oil) than animal fats (butter, cheese, milk, cream).

Fat does not have much effect on your blood glucose, but too much of the wrong kinds of fat will raise your blood cholesterol.

Fats are found in:

- oils

- butter and margarine

- olives

- cream, sour cream and cream cheese

- nuts and seeds

- salad dressings and mayonnaise

- whole and 2% milk, cheese (except skim milk and fat-free cheese) and fatty meats

- desserts, sweets, snack foods (such as chips and crackers), fried foods, gravies and sauces.

What are the different kinds of fats?

There are four main kinds of fats in foods:

Check nutrition labels for saturated and trans fats. Avoid these foods if you can.

- saturated fats

- trans fats

- polyunsaturated fats (omega-3 fatty acids are a type of polyunsaturated fat)

- monounsaturated fats

Are some fats better for me than others?

Yes. Too many saturated and trans fats will raise your "bad" cholesterol, or LDL. These can be found in fatty meats and dairy products, stick margarine, shortening, butter, lard, snack foods, sweets and desserts, fried foods, fast foods, and foods that contain hydrogenated, partially-hydrogenated or tropical oils (palm, coconut or palm kernel oil). **Eat as few saturated and trans fats as possible.**

Monounsaturated fats will lower your "bad" cholesterol, or LDL. They can also help raise your "good" cholesterol, or HDL. Sources of monounsaturated fats include olive oil, peanut oil, canola oil, olives, avocados, nuts and seeds.

Polyunsaturated fats will also lower your "bad" cholesterol, or LDL. Sources of polyunsaturated fats include tub, liquid and spray margarines; mayonnaise; salad dressings; and nuts and seeds.

Omega-3 fatty acids are found in salmon, albacore tuna, herring, mackerel, sardines and rainbow trout. Omega-3 fatty acids can raise your "good" cholesterol, or HDL. They can also lower the amount of fat (triglycerides) in your blood. Try to eat two or more meals of fatty fish a week. Other sources of omega-3 fatty acids include soy and canola oil, black walnuts, flax and flaxseed oil. (See table at the end of this chapter.)

Fish oil and flax seed oil both contain omega-3 fatty acids.

What is cholesterol?

Cholesterol is a fatty substance made in the body by the liver. It also comes from some of the foods you eat.

What foods contain cholesterol?

Cholesterol is found only in animal products, including:

- high-fat dairy products (whole and 2% milk, cheese, cream, butter and ice cream)

- beef, pork, lamb, veal and other meats

- chicken, turkey and other poultry

- fish and other seafood

- egg yolks.

How can I cut back on the unhealthy fats and cholesterol in my foods?

To reduce fat and cholesterol:

- Choose fish, poultry with the skin removed and lean red meats with the fat trimmed off. Keep the total amount of cooked meat to 6 ounces or less each day. (Three ounces of meat is about the size of a deck of cards or the palm of your hand.)

- Choose lean cuts of beef—such as top round, top loin, round tip, eye of round, sirloin, tenderloin and ground beef—that are 15 percent fat or less.

Choose lean meats, and always trim the fat off.

- Choose lean cuts of pork, such as loin chops and roasts, butterfly chops, sirloin chops and tenderloin.

- Choose any cuts of lamb or veal except shoulder roasts and chops.

- Use low-fat cooking methods such as broiling, roasting, grilling, steaming, stir-frying and microwaving.

- Make sandwiches with fresh vegetables along with one or two slices of lower-fat deli meats, such as roast beef, ham, Canadian bacon, sliced turkey or chicken.

- Choose low-fat or fat-free yogurt and sour cream in dressings and desserts.

- Use 1% or skim milk.

- Choose low-fat or fat-free cheeses, such as cottage cheese, ricotta, farmers or skim-milk mozzarella. Choose reduced-fat varieties of Swiss, cheddar, American and Colby cheeses.

- Cook and bake in non-stick cookware, or use a non-stick vegetable spray.

- Choose fat-free sauces and dressings.

- Eat no more than three to four egg yolks per week.

For more information, see the table at the end of this chapter.

If you cook with non-stick pans, you only need to use a tiny bit of oil to sauté foods. Better yet, try adding vegetable broth instead.

Vitamins, minerals and water

All foods contain vitamins, minerals and water. These provide no calories and have no effect on your blood glucose levels.

Should I take vitamin and mineral supplements?

Eating a variety of foods from all food groups will help you to get the right amount of vitamins and minerals in your diet. But some people may need additional vitamins or minerals. Your dietitian will review your diet and health history to see if you need to take supplements.

How much salt (sodium) should I eat?

For good health, you should try to eat no more than 2,300 mg of sodium a day. (One teaspoon of regular table salt has about 2,300 mg of sodium.) If you have high blood pressure, you should try to eat less than 1,500 mg of sodium a day.

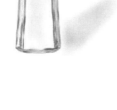

The following foods are naturally low in sodium:

- fresh fruits and vegetables

- unprocessed beef, pork, lamb, chicken, turkey, cornish hen, fish, seafood

- eggs

- fresh tofu

- unsalted dried peas and beans

- unsalted nuts and seeds

- plain grains

- plain milk, plain yogurt

- oils.

How can I cut back on the amount of sodium I eat?

Try not to use salt in cooking or at the table. Perk up your foods with pepper, vinegar, lemon, salt-free herbs and spices, and other seasonings.

Try to avoid foods that are high in sodium, including:

- processed and convenience foods (snack foods; canned, frozen and other packaged foods; processed meats and cheeses)

- condiments (ketchup, mustard, soy sauce, pickles, olives)

- restaurant and fast foods.

When you eat out, ask for your meal to be made without salt whenever possible.

Sodium is in many store-bought sauces, soups, condiments and canned vegetables. Check nutrition labels to see how much sodium is in your food.

How much water should I drink?

Honor your thirst. Drink water and other calorie-free drinks to quench your thirst as you need it.

Food planning

At this point you may wonder, "So what *can* I eat?" Your dietitian will create a meal plan based on your:

- blood glucose goals

- cholesterol levels

- body weight

- blood pressure

- medicines

- usual eating habits

- activity level.

Food-planning tools include:

Your dietitian will work with you to decide what method of food planning is best for you.

- **My Pyramid.** This guide is offered by the US government. It advises staying active, limiting calories and eating healthy foods.

- **Carb counting.** Counting carbohydrates is a great way to add variety to your food plan. Simply track how many "units" of carbohydrate you have each day.

- **Exchanges.** This system groups foods based on the amounts of carbohydrate, protein and fat they contain.

For more information on food planning, go to chapter 10, "Your Diabetes Care Plan."

What are the nutrition facts labels on food packages?

A nutrition facts label will tell you how many calories and nutrients are in one serving of that food. Below is a sample nutrition facts label.

Nutrition Facts

Serving Size ½ cup (90g)

Servings Per Container 4

Amount Per Serving

Calories 100	Calories from Fat 30

	% Daily Value
Total Fat 3g	5%
Saturated Fat 0g	0%
Trans Fat 0g	
Cholesterol 0mg	0%
Sodium 300mg	13%
Total Carbohydrate 13g	4%
Dietary Fiber 3g	12%
Sugars 3g	
Protein 3g	

Vitamin A	0%	•	Vitamin C	0%
Calcium	0%	•	Iron	3%

*Percent Daily Values are based on a 2,000 calorie diet. Your daily values may be higher or lower depending on your calorie needs:

	Calories:	2,000	2,500
Total Fat	Less than	65g	80g
Sat Fat	Less than	20g	25g
Cholesterol	Less than	300mg	300mg
Sodium	Less than	2,400mg	2,400mg
Total Carbohydrate		300g	375g
Dietary Fiber		25g	30g

Serving size

When counting calories and other nutrients, you need to know how many servings you are eating.

Check the serving size, then compare this to the amount on your plate.

Check the serving size carefully. This tells you how large one serving will be. Then, look at the servings per container to check how many servings are in each package. Even a small package can have more than one serving. If you eat two servings, you will get twice the number of calories and nutrients listed on the label.

Calories

Both the total number of calories and the number of calories from fat are listed. No more than 30% of your total calories should come from fat.

Total fat

Total fat includes all the saturated, polyunsaturated, monounsaturated and trans fats in one serving. Try to avoid saturated and trans fats. These can raise your cholesterol.

Cholesterol

Limit the amount of cholesterol you eat to help lower the amount of cholesterol in your blood. You should eat no more than 200 to 300 mg of cholesterol a day.

Sodium

You should limit the amount of sodium (salt) that you eat to no more than 2,300 mg per day. If you have high blood pressure, you should eat no more than 1,500 mg per day.

Total carbohydrate

Since carbohydrates have the greatest effect on your blood glucose, it is very important to track how many carbohydrates you are eating. The amount of carbohydrate on a food label is always listed as "Total Carbohydrate." This includes the amount of carbohydrate that comes from sugar.

Dietary fiber

Fiber is important for good health, but it does not affect your blood glucose. Try to eat at least 20 to 35 grams a day.

Sugars

This number includes both sugars that occur naturally in the food and sugars that have been added to the food.

There are many names for sugar, including corn syrup, high-fructose corn syrup, maltose, dextrose, sucrose, fructose, lactose and honey.

Protein

Note the amount of protein listed to help you stay within your daily protein guidelines. Your dietitian will tell you how much protein is right for you.

Artificial Sweeteners

Five artificial sweeteners have been approved for use by the Food and Drug Administration (FDA) in the United States. None of them has any calories. All are safe to use.

Acesulfame K (Sunette and Sweet One): 200 times sweeter than sugar. For table use and cooking.

Aspartame (NutraSweet and Equal): 200 times sweeter than sugar. For table use and in cold foods only (not for cooking).

Saccharin (Sugar Twin, Sweet 10, Sweet 'N' Low, Sucaryl and Featherweight): 300 times sweeter than sugar. For table use and cooking.

Sucralose (Splenda): 600 times sweeter than sugar. For table use and cooking.

Neotame: 7,000 to 13,000 times sweeter than sugar. Used in prepared foods.

Sugar Alcohols

Like artificial sweeteners, sugar alcohols are safe to use. But too much sugar alcohol can cause diarrhea (loose stools) in some people.

Sugar alcohols have about 2 calories per gram, so they can raise blood glucose. Common sugar alcohols include sorbitol, mannitol, xylitol, isomalt, lactitol, maltitol, erythritol and hydrogenated starch hydrolysate.

Remember: "Sugar-free" does not mean "carbohydrate-free." Always check the total carbohydrate on the nutrition facts label.

How can I eat healthy when eating away from home?

It is easier to plan healthy meals when you cook at home than when you eat out. When you eat out, try to make healthy choices about what you eat and how much you eat. The following tips can help make eating out healthier and more enjoyable.

- **Know your meal plan.**

- **Plan ahead.** If you can, plan where you will eat, what you will eat and how much you will eat.

- **Know your usual portion sizes.** Practice measuring foods at home so that you can judge portion sizes when you are away from home.

- **Ask how foods have been prepared if you are uncertain.** Choose foods that are grilled, broiled or baked. Avoid fried foods.

- **Ask for sauces, condiments, gravies, dressings and similar foods to be served "on the side."** This lets you control how much you use.

- **Ask for reduced-calorie foods whenever possible,** such as sugar-free syrup or low-fat or no-fat salad dressing. They may not appear on the menu, but many restaurants will serve them to you if you ask for them.

Think about skipping the appetizers. They are often high in fat, salt and cholesterol.

- **Ask for your foods to be prepared without added salt if possible.**

Some restaurants will let you order half portions.

- **Don't overeat.** Restaurants are known to serve large portions. Think about splitting your meal with someone else or taking the leftovers home for another meal. You may want to ask your server for a carry-out container at the beginning of the meal. Pack up half of the meal right away to help reduce the temptation to overeat.

- **Be careful of salad bars and all-you-can-eat buffets.** Calories add up very quickly.

Remember, the more you know about food and portion sizes, the easier it will be to manage your diabetes while eating out.

What about alcohol?

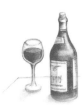

Alcohol's effect on your blood glucose will vary. It will depend on what you drink, how much you drink and whether you have eaten any food. For information on alcohol and blood glucose, see chapter 8, "Day-to-Day Living."

Body Mass Index Table (*for adults only*)

Height	60"	62"	64"	66"	68"	70"	72"	74"	76"	78"	80"
Weight											
100	20	18	17	16	15	14	14	13	12	12	11
105	21	19	18	17	16	15	14	14	13	12	12
110	22	20	19	18	17	16	15	14	13	13	12
115	23	21	20	19	18	17	16	15	14	13	13
120	23	22	21	19	18	17	16	15	14	14	13
125	24	23	22	20	19	18	17	16	15	14	14
130	25	24	22	21	20	19	18	17	16	15	14
135	26	25	23	22	21	19	18	17	16	16	15
140	27	26	24	23	21	20	19	18	17	16	15
145	28	27	25	23	22	21	20	19	18	17	16
150	29	27	26	24	23	22	20	19	18	17	17
155	30	28	27	25	24	22	21	20	19	18	17
160	31	29	28	26	24	23	22	21	20	19	18
165	32	30	28	27	25	24	22	21	20	19	18
170	33	31	29	27	26	24	23	22	21	20	19
175	34	32	30	28	27	25	24	23	21	20	19
180	35	33	31	29	27	26	24	23	22	21	20
185	36	34	32	30	28	27	25	24	23	21	20
190	37	35	33	31	29	27	26	24	23	22	21
195	38	36	34	32	30	28	27	25	24	23	21
200	39	37	34	32	30	29	27	26	24	23	22
205	40	38	35	33	31	29	28	26	25	24	23
210	41	38	36	34	32	30	29	27	26	24	23
215	42	39	37	35	33	31	29	28	26	25	24
220	43	40	38	36	34	32	30	28	27	25	24
225	44	41	39	36	34	32	30	29	27	26	25
230	45	42	40	37	35	33	31	30	28	27	25
235	46	43	40	38	36	34	32	30	29	27	26
240	47	44	41	39	37	35	33	31	29	28	26
245	48	45	42	40	37	35	33	32	30	28	27
250	49	46	43	40	38	36	34	32	30	29	28
255	50	47	44	41	39	37	35	33	31	30	28
260	51	48	45	42	40	37	35	33	32	30	29
265	52	49	46	43	40	38	36	34	32	31	29
270	53	49	46	44	41	39	37	35	33	31	30
275	54	50	47	44	42	40	37	35	34	32	30
280	55	51	48	45	43	40	38	36	34	32	31
285	56	52	49	46	43	41	39	37	35	33	31
290	57	53	50	47	44	42	39	37	35	34	32
295	58	54	51	48	45	42	40	38	36	34	32
300	59	55	52	49	46	43	41	39	37	35	33

white = healthy weight   light gray = overweight   dark gray = obese

Sources of Omega-3 Fatty Acids

Food	Omega-3 fatty acids
Mackerel (3 ounces)	0.34–1.57 grams
Chinook salmon (3 ounces)	1.48 grams
Atlantic salmon, farmed (3 ounces)	1.09–1.83 grams
Herring (3 ounces)	1.71–1.81 grams
White tuna, canned in water, drained (3 ounces)	0.73 grams
Anchovy (3 ounces)	1.2 grams
Sockeye salmon (3 ounces)	0.68 grams
Coho salmon (3 ounces)	0.94 grams
Pink salmon (3 ounces)	1.09 grams
Halibut (3 ounces)	0.4–1.0 grams
Rainbow trout, farmed (3 ounces)	0.98 grams
Flaxseed (1 tablespoon)	2.2 grams
Flaxseed oil (1 tablespoon)	8.5 grams
English walnuts (1 tablespoon)	0.7 grams
Canola oil (1 tablespoon)	1.3 grams
Soybean oil (1 tablespoon)	0.9 grams

Calories and Fat in 3 Ounces of Cooked Meat

	Calories	Total fat (g)	Saturated fat (g)	Cholesterol (mg)
Lean cuts of meat (3 ounces)				
Beef eye round	143	4.2	1.5	59
Beef top round	153	4.2	1.4	71
Beef tip round	157	5.9	2.1	69
Beef top sirloin	165	6.1	2.4	76
Beef top loin	176	8.0	3.1	65
Beef tenderloin	179	8.5	3.2	71
Beef flank	176	8.6	3.7	57
Lean cuts of pork (3 ounces)				
Pork tenderloin	139	4.1	1.4	67
Pork boneless sirloin chop	164	5.7	1.9	78
Pork boneless top loin roast	165	6.1	2.2	66
Pork boneless top loin chop	173	6.6	2.3	68
Pork loin chop	172	6.9	2.5	70
Pork rib chop	186	8.3	2.9	69
Pork boneless rib roast	182	8.6	3.0	71
Pork sirloin roast	184	8.7	3.1	73

Calories and Fat in 3 Ounces of Cooked Meat *(continued)*

	Calories	Total fat (g)	Saturated fat (g)	Cholesterol (mg)
Ground meat products (3 ounces)				
Low-fat ground beef	149	7	2.7	64
Ground beef – 95% lean	132	5	2.0	66
Ground beef – 90% lean	169	9	3.5	70
Ground beef – 85% lean	204	12	4.7	71
Ground beef – 80% lean	228	15	5.9	74
Ground pork – 80% lean	252	18	6.6	80
Ground turkey	195	12	4.7	59
Skinless chicken (3 ounces)				
Chicken breast	140	3.0	0.9	72
Chicken leg	162	7.2	2.0	80
Chicken thigh	178	9.3	2.6	81
Fish (3 ounces)				
Cod	89	0.7	0.1	47
Flounder	62	1.3	0.3	58
Halibut	119	2.5	0.4	35
Orange roughy	75	0.8	0.0	22
Shrimp	84	0.9	0.2	166

Fiber Content of Selected Foods

Food	Amount	Fiber (grams)
Apple with skin	1 medium	3.5
Banana	1 medium	2.4
Cantaloupe	¼ melon	1.0
Cherries, sweet	10	1.2
Peach with skin	1 medium	1.9
Pear with skin	½ large	3.1
Prunes	3	3.0
Raisins	¼ cup	3.1
Raspberries	½ cup	3.1
Strawberries	1 cup	3.0
Orange	1 medium	2.6
Prune juice	½ cup	1.3
Celery, diced	½ cup raw	1.1
Cucumber	½ cup raw	0.4
Lettuce	1 cup raw	0.9
Mushrooms	½ cups raw	0.9
Tomato	1 medium raw	1.5
Spinach	1 cup raw	1.2
Asparagus	½ cup cooked	1.0

Fiber Content of Selected Foods *(continued)*

Food	Amount	Fiber (grams)
Green beans	½ cup cooked	1.6
Broccoli	½ cup cooked	2.2
Brussels sprouts	½ cup cooked	2.3
Parsnips	½ cup cooked	2.7
Potato with skin	1 medium	2.5
Spinach	½ cup cooked	2.1
Sweet potato	½ medium	1.7
Turnip	½ cup cooked	1.6
Zucchini	½ cup cooked	1.8
Almonds	10	1.1
Peanuts	10	1.4
Popcorn	1 cup popped	1.0
All-bran cereal	⅓ cup	8.5
Bran Buds	⅓ cup	7.9
Bran Chex	⅔ cup	4.6
Corn Bran	⅔ cup	5.4
40% bran cereal	¾ cup	4.0
Raisin Bran	¾ cup	4.0

Fiber Content of Selected Foods *(continued)*

Food	Amount	Fiber (grams)
Shredded Wheat	⅔ cup	2.6
Oatmeal, all types	¾ cup cooked	1.6
Cornflakes	1¼ cups	0.3
Baked beans	½ cup cooked	8.8
Dried peas	½ cup cooked	4.7
Kidney beans	½ cup cooked	7.3
Lima beans	½ cup cooked	4.5
Lentils	½ cup cooked	3.7
Navy beans	½ cup cooked	6.0
Bagels	1 bagel	0.6
Bran muffins	1 muffin	2.5
French bread	1 slice	0.7
Oatmeal bread	1 slice	0.5
Pumpernickel bread	1 slice	1.0
Whole wheat bread	1 slice	1.4
Brown rice	½ cup cooked	1.0
Spaghetti	½ cup cooked	1.1
Whole wheat flour	½ cup uncooked	6.9

Chapter 6

Staying Active

➤ Physical activity may be the best thing you can to do manage diabetes and improve your health. This is true no matter your age or fitness level.

➤ If exercise is new to you, it's important to set realistic goals for yourself.

➤ To prevent injury, it helps to warm up before exercise and cool down afterward.

➤ If you take certain medicines, you will need to take steps to prevent hypoglycemia (low blood glucose) before and after exercise.

➤ Work with your diabetes care team to find an exercise plan that's safe for you.

It's never too late to become more active.

Exercise is good for everyone, whether or not you have diabetes. It can help you lose weight, improve your health and make you feel better. If you have diabetes, exercise can also help control your blood glucose and reduce your risk of heart disease.

No matter your age or fitness level, research shows that becoming more active can make you healthier and improve your quality of life.

Why should I exercise?

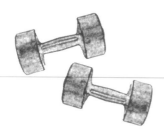

Because exercise:

- lowers blood glucose and helps your body use insulin better

- lowers cholesterol and triglycerides (fats in the blood), raises "good" cholesterol (HDL) and lowers blood pressure

- increases strength, endurance, flexibility and balance; gives you more energy

- increases the rate at which you use energy, which helps you lose fat and gain muscle

- helps build strong bones, muscles and joints—and keeps them healthy

- helps you control your weight

- reduces stress, makes you feel better

- may reduce how much medicine you need.

Before You Begin

- Get a medical check-up. Talk to your doctor about which activities are safe for you. You may need to see a specialist if you have not exercised in a long time or if you have certain health problems. Your doctor can suggest a specialist if needed.

- Talk with your diabetes care team about a plan. You may need to adjust your medicine as you become more active.

How do I get started?

Choose one or more activities that you enjoy. If it is hard to exercise because of arthritis or other joint problems, try swimming, water aerobics, chair exercises or other exercise that increases your heart rate without stressing your joints.

Make sure that what you do is right for your level of fitness. Start slowly and do more only as you are able.

Walking is often a good way to get started. It is easy and cheap. All you need are good socks and a pair of supportive shoes that fit well. Change your shoes often, if you use them regularly, and plan to buy a new pair at least twice a year for good support.

Checking your blood glucose level before and after exercise is a great way to see the immediate benefits you are getting.

What kinds of exercise should I do?

Talk to your doctor before starting any exercise program.

You can benefit from four basic kinds of physical activity.

- Aerobic exercise, for your heart and lungs

- Strength and endurance training, for strength and balance

- Flexibility (stretching) exercises, for limber joints and muscles

- General activity throughout the day, for burning calories and staying fit

Aerobic (heart and lung) exercise

Activities that make you breathe harder and keep your heart rate up for several minutes at a time will improve your aerobic (heart and lung) fitness.

Aerobic exercise does not have to take great effort. Start slowly, doing something you enjoy. Work up to a harder pace over time.

Examples of aerobic exercise include:

- brisk walking

- stair climbing

- swimming

- water aerobics

- dancing

- hiking

- cycling

- using a stationary bicycle

- taking an aerobics class

- basketball

- volleyball

- tennis, squash, racquetball

- cross-country skiing.

Try to do aerobic exercise at least 5 times a week. Start slowly, exercising for longer periods of time as you are able.

How much aerobic exercise should I do?

Try to do some type of aerobic exercise at least 5 days a week for 30 minutes or more.

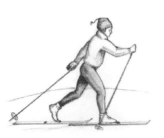

Other tips for aerobic fitness:

- You can begin exercising for as few as 5 minutes at a time. Exercise for longer periods of time as you are able.

- You can break your exercise into 10-minute segments.

Always warm up before exercise and cool down after. This will help prevent injury.

- To prevent injury, warm up for 5 to 10 minutes, then stretch your muscles and joints for several minutes before exercising.

- To prevent injury, stretch and cool down for at least 5 to 10 minutes after exercising.

- You are more likely to lose weight if you exercise for at least 30 minutes without stopping.

How hard should I exercise?

Studies show that moderate exercise—not too light, but not too hard—is best for people with diabetes. How can you tell if you are getting moderate exercise? One way to tell is the "talk test."

The "talk test" is simple. If you have enough breath to sing while exercising, then you are doing light exercise. If you do not have enough breath to sing, but you have enough to talk easily with another person, then you are doing moderate exercise. If you are too winded or out of breath to talk with another person, you are doing hard exercise.

Strength and endurance training

Muscles get stronger when you move them against a force, such as a weight or elastic band. This is called **strength training.** Muscles are able to work longer when you move them over and over in the same way. This is called **endurance training.**

Studies show that strength training is safe and effective for women and men of all ages, even those who are not in perfect health. It can improve blood glucose and help prevent problems from diabetes, especially when combined with aerobic exercise. It can also improve endurance and balance.

Examples of strength training include:

- hand weights

- elastic bands

- weight machines

- stair climbing.

You should get expert advice about how best to do strength training. You can be injured if you do not use proper form and technique. Warming up and stretching before you exercise and cooling down and stretching after you exercise will help prevent injury.

Lifting weights just two or three times a week can make your muscles bigger and stronger.

Before you start any strength training program, get your doctor's approval—especially if you have high blood pressure, retinopathy, heart disease, nerve damage or kidney disease.

How often should I do strength training?

For best results, do strength training at least twice a week, but no more than every other day. Your muscles need a day to rest between workouts.

The type of strength training you choose will depend on your goals.

In general, you should try to do each exercise 8 to 12 times without stopping. These 8 to 12 repetitions, or "reps," are called a set. Try to do 2 sets, resting briefly in between.

Flexibility

Stretching helps to keep your joints flexible and reduce your chances of injury. Stretching muscles and joints when they are cold and stiff can injure them, so take a few minutes to warm up before you stretch.

An easy way to warm up is to walk while swinging your arms in wide circles. Warm up for at least 5 to 10 minutes before stretching.

Start each stretch slowly, breathing out slowly as you gently stretch the muscle. Try to hold each stretch for at least 20 to 30 seconds.

Avoid These Stretching Mistakes

Don't bounce when you stretch. That is, don't use your weight or the motion of your body to stretch farther than is comfortable for you. Stretch slowly, as far as you can without causing pain, then hold the stretch. This does a better job of stretching the muscles and joints and is less likely to injure you.

Don't stretch a muscle that is not warmed up.

Don't hold your breath. Breathe naturally as you stretch.

More hints:

- Try doing a few stretches right after a shower or when soaking in a hot tub. The hot water will warm your muscles, making them easier to stretch.

- Do a few simple stretches before getting out of bed in the morning. Stretch your entire body by pointing your toes and reaching your arms above your head.

- Join a stretching, yoga or tai chi class. This may help you to stay on a regular stretching program.

Some people like to stretch right after they get out of the shower, while their muscles are still warm.

How often should I stretch?

Try to stretch at least 3 times per week.

Being active throughout the day

Even fidgeting can help you burn calories!

Any kind of **physical activity** throughout the day will help you burn calories and keep fit. Whenever you can, take the stairs instead of the elevator, park your car at the far end of the parking lot, and walk instead of drive.

Always look for new ways to increase your daily activity: walk farther, climb more stairs, tidy up your home or office.

Here are more ways to increase your daily activity:

- Play with your kids or grandkids inside and outside.

- Walk the dog.

Try not to sit still for more than 30 minutes at a time.

- Use a push mower instead of a riding mower.

- Garden in the summer.

- Rake the leaves in the fall.

- Shovel the snow from your driveway and sidewalks.

- Stretch, walk in place or do jumping jacks while you watch TV. Get up and be active during commercials.

- Try to not sit for more than two hours total per day.

- If you live in an apartment building, walk in the hallways and use the stairs every day.

- Walk around while you talk on the phone.

- Wash your own car.

- Take the bus. Get off before your stop and walk the rest of the way home.

- Walk whenever you can, such as in airports while waiting for your plane, when shopping, or just for the fun of it!

- Clean your house or your office.

- Walk with co-workers at lunch.

- Use the stairs instead of the elevator. Walk up more flights of stairs as you are able.

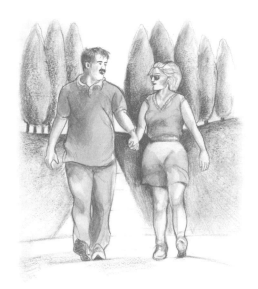

Use the chart on the next page to see how many calories you burn with common activities. Note: this chart is for a person who weighs 150 pounds. The more you weigh, the more calories you will use doing the same activity.

For example, a 100-pound person will use a third fewer calories than a person weighing 150 pounds. A 200-pound person will use a third more calories.

Exercising harder or faster will increase the calories you use a little bit. A better way to burn more calories is to exercise for a longer period of time.

Calories Spent in Various Exercises

Activity	Calories per hour
Light activity	
Light housework	150
Strolling (1 mile per hour)	150
Golf, using cart	175
Level walking (2 miles per hour)	200
Moderate activity	
Cycling (5.5 miles per hour)	210
Gardening	220
Canoeing (2.5 miles per hour)	230
Cleaning windows, mopping, vacuuming	240
Lawn mowing with a power mower	250
Lawn mowing with a push mower	270
Walking (3 miles per hour)	275
Bowling	300
Golf, pulling cart	300
Scrubbing floors	300
Rowboating (2.5 miles per hour)	300
Swimming (0.25 miles per hour)	300
Cycling (8 miles per hour)	325
Golf, carrying clubs	350

Calories Spent in Various Exercises *(continued)*

Activity	Calories per hour
Badminton	350
Square dancing	350
Doubles tennis	360
Calisthenics and ballet exercises	360
Table tennis	360
Walking (4 miles per hour)	360

Strenuous activity

Activity	Calories per hour
Vigorous dancing	320–500
Cycling (10 miles per hour)	400
Ice skating (10 miles per hour)	400
Ditch digging, hand shovel	400
Wood chopping or sawing	400–600
Walking (5 miles per hour)	420
Cycling (11 miles per hour)	420
Singles tennis	420
Jogging (5 miles per hour)	480
Hill climbing (100 feet per hour)	490
Downhill skiing	550
Squash and handball	600
Cross-country skiing	600–1,200
Running (10 miles per hour)	900

Safe Exercise

Start slowly—exercise just 5 to 10 minutes a day if you have been very inactive.

Wear comfortable, supportive shoes and polyester or cotton-polyester blend socks. Check your feet after exercise for blisters, calluses or other signs of poor fit or injury. Tell your doctor if you have any problems.

Wear or carry identification (ID) that shows you have diabetes.

Drink water and other fluids before, during and after exercise. Honor your thirst!

If you take certain medicines (insulin, sulfonylureas or meglitinides) it is important to take steps to prevent hypoglycemia (low blood glucose).

- Do not exercise when your insulin is "peaking" (working at its strongest level).

- Be aware that low blood glucose can occur several hours, or even a day, after exercise.

- Check your blood glucose before exercising.
  - **If your glucose level is 60 or less:** Eat or drink 15 grams of carbohydrate. Wait 15 minutes, then check your blood glucose again before exercising. If it is still low, eat another 15 grams of carbohydrate until your blood glucose is normal. (See next page for a list of foods with 15 grams of carbohydrate.)

- **If your glucose level is between 60 and 100:** Have a snack with 15 grams of carbohydrate before you exercise.

- **If your glucose level is between 100 and 150:** You may need a snack with 15 grams of carbohydrate after you exercise.

- **If your glucose is over 300:** Exercise can make your blood glucose go even higher. Do not exercise until your blood glucose is lower.

• Check your blood glucose after you exercise.

• In general, you should eat or drink 15 grams of carbohydrate for every hour that you exercise.

• Take a carbohydrate snack with you when you exercise. Here are some examples of snacks that have 15 grams of carbohydrate:

   4-ounce juice box

   1 small box of raisins (about 2 tablespoons)

   3 to 4 glucose tablets

   1 small piece of fruit

   8 ounces of a sports drink

   4 to 6 crackers.

• The longer and harder you exercise, the more likely you are to need extra carbohydrates later. Test your blood glucose several hours after exercise to check for delayed hypoglycemia.

Chapter 7

Preventing Problems and Reducing Your Risks from Diabetes

➤ Having diabetes puts you at greater risk for many health problems, including heart attack, stroke, kidney failure, nerve damage and blindness.

➤ The good news is, you can avoid most of these problems by doing three simple things:

- Control your blood glucose.

- Control your blood pressure.

- Control your cholesterol.

➤ You will need to do all that you can to avoid infections. Infections will raise your blood glucose. And high blood glucose will make infections more likely to occur.

Over time, high blood glucose, blood pressure and cholesterol can damage many parts of the body, including the heart, blood vessels, nerves, eyes and kidneys. Damage to large blood vessels can lead to heart attack and stroke. Damage to small blood vessels can cause kidney disease, eye problems and nerve damage.

The good news is that people with both type 1 and type 2 diabetes can prevent or delay complications. How? By managing blood glucose, blood pressure and cholesterol.

Taking care of your heart and blood vessels

The heart and blood vessels make up the **cardiovascular system** (cardio = heart; vascular = blood vessels). The heart pumps blood through large blood vessels called **arteries**. Other blood vessels called **veins** carry blood back to the heart.

If your blood vessels are thick, hard and rigid, we say you have arteriosclerosis.

High blood glucose, blood pressure and cholesterol can damage blood vessels, causing them to become thick, hard and rigid. This raises your risk of having a heart attack or stroke.

What is high blood pressure (hypertension)?

Blood pressure is the force of your blood pressing against the walls of your arteries. It is measured with two numbers, written as a fraction: for example, 130/80, which is read as "130 over 80."

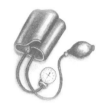

Anyone can have high blood pressure (hypertension). But often you can't feel high blood pressure, which is why many people don't know they have it.

High blood pressure is common in people who have diabetes.

- It may cause up to 75 percent of heart disease in people with diabetes.

- Just having diabetes makes you 2 to 4 times more likely to have a heart attack or stroke.

- High blood pressure also raises your risk of developing kidney and eye problems.

To lower these risks, it is important to control your blood pressure.

Blood Pressure Readings

The first, and higher, number is your "systolic" blood pressure. The systolic number measures the pressure in your arteries as your heart beats.

The second, and lower, number is the "diastolic" blood pressure. The diastolic number measures the resting pressure in your arteries between the beats of your heart.

What is high cholesterol?

Cholesterol is measured in three different ways: total cholesterol, LDL (or "bad" cholesterol) and HDL (or "good" cholesterol).

If your cholesterol is too high, the insides of your large blood vessels can narrow and become clogged. This makes it harder for blood and oxygen to get to all parts of your body. Your doctor should check your blood cholesterol and triglycerides (blood fats) at least once a year.

How does diabetes affect my heart and blood vessels?

High blood glucose levels can cause your arteries to become stiff, or to lose their ability to stretch. When this happens, your blood pressure goes up.

Over time, high blood pressure can cause the walls of your arteries to get thicker and rougher, making the opening of the arteries smaller and allowing less blood to flow through. This makes it easier for fat, cholesterol and other sticky materials (called **plaque**) to build up inside the artery walls.

Cholesterol Goals

Total cholesterol.................... Less than 200

HDL ("good") cholesterol..... Over 40 for men; over 50 for women

LDL ("bad") cholesterol........ Under 100 (under 70 if you already have heart disease)

Triglycerides.......................... Under 150

As plaque builds up on the artery walls, there is even less room for blood to flow. Sometimes, a piece of this plaque will break off and completely block the flow of blood.

If your blood vessels are narrowed and clogged, we say you have atherosclerosis.

- **A blocked brain artery causes stroke.** Common warning signs include:
  - Sudden numbness or weakness in the face, arm or leg (often on one side of the body)
  - Sudden confusion or trouble understanding what is going on
  - Sudden trouble seeing in one or both eyes
  - Sudden trouble speaking, understanding speech, or reading
  - Sudden trouble walking, loss of balance, dizziness or problems with coordination
  - Sudden, severe headache with no known cause.

- **A blocked heart artery causes heart attack.** Symptoms may go away, then come back. The most common warning signs include:
  - Pain, pressure, tightness, squeezing or burning in one side of the chest, the middle of the chest or between the shoulder blades
  - Pain or pressure that spreads to the shoulders, arms, neck or jaw

- Fainting or feeling lightheaded, usually with other symptoms

- Heartburn or feeling sick to your stomach, usually with other symptoms

- Cold sweats or heavy sweating

- Feeling very tired or more tired than normal

- Shortness of breath

- Sudden, strong anxiety.

Like heart attack and stroke, peripheral artery disease is more common in people with diabetes.

- Poor blood flow and blockage can also occur in your lower legs. This is called **peripheral artery disease.** For a list of symptoms, see page 112.

What can I do to prevent heart disease and stroke?

- Keep your blood pressure below 130/80. If you take blood pressure medicine, take it every day as prescribed by your doctor.

- Have your blood pressure checked every time you visit your doctor or clinic. If you have high blood pressure, you may be asked to check your blood pressure at home.

- Eat a healthy, well-balanced diet (see chapter 5).

- Control your blood glucose. Aim for an A1c of less than 7%.

- If you take medicine to lower cholesterol, take it every day as your doctor tells you.

- Keep your total cholesterol less than 200.

- Keep your LDL cholesterol less than 100. If you have heart disease, your LDL should be less than 70.

- Keep your HDL over 40 if you are a man and over 50 if you are a woman.

- Keep your triglycerides below 150.

- Limit alcohol to one drink per day if you are a woman and two drinks a day if you are a man.

- Exercise regularly. Get at least 30 minutes of exercise on most days of the week.

- Maintain a healthy weight.

- Pay attention to how stress affects you.

- Avoid smoking and using tobacco.

- Take an aspirin every day if your doctor tells you to.

Think of LDL as "lousy cholesterol" and HDL as "healthy cholesterol."

Taking care of your kidneys

The job of your kidneys is to filter waste and extra water from your blood and get rid of it as urine. Your kidneys are always "cleaning" your blood. You can take care of your kidneys by keeping your blood glucose and blood pressure as close to normal as possible.

Your doctor will test your urine once a year to make sure your kidneys are working properly.

What is kidney disease?

Your kidneys have many small blood vessels that can be damaged by high blood glucose and high blood pressure. When these blood vessels are damaged, your kidneys may not filter waste out of your blood.

Nephropathy is another name for kidney disease.

When this happens, waste can build up in your blood. Also, important nutrients such as protein that should stay in the blood can start to leak out into your urine. Protein in the urine is one of the first signs of kidney disease.

You are at higher risk for getting kidney disease if your blood glucose and blood pressure are not well controlled.

What can I do to prevent or treat kidney disease?

- Keep your blood pressure below 130/80. If you take blood pressure medicine, be sure to take it every day as prescribed by your doctor. Have your blood pressure checked every time you visit your doctor or clinic.

- Tell your doctor at once if:
  - you often feel the urge to urinate.
  - it hurts when you urinate.
  - your urine is bloody or cloudy.
  - you have back pain, chills or fever.

  These are signs that your bladder may be infected. Frequent bladder infections may cause kidney disease.

- Blood pressure medicines called "ACE inhibitors" or "ARBs" can sometimes slow kidney disease in people with diabetes. Ask your doctor about these medicines.

- Keep your blood glucose in your target range. If you take diabetes medicine, take it every day as your doctor has prescribed. Write the results in your record book or journal so you can keep track.

Don't wait to treat a bladder infection. Bladder infections can lead to kidney disease. If you have any symptoms, see your doctor.

- Try to keep your A1c below 7%. Make sure your doctor checks your A1c at least twice a year.

- If you smoke, ask your care provider for help with quitting.

- Have your urine tested once a year for protein. Protein in the urine is often the first sign of kidney disease.

- Follow a healthy, well-balanced, low-sodium diet. Ask your dietitian to help you with your meal plan.

Diabetes and Kidney Disease

As many as one in ten people with type 2 diabetes and four in ten people with type 1 diabetes will get kidney disease.

One in four of all new cases of kidney failure occur in people who have diabetes.

Fortunately, most people with diabetes will not have kidney disease severe enough to cause their kidneys to fail.

Taking care of your nerves

Your nerves are like a telephone system, carrying messages from your brain to all parts of your body and then back to your brain again.

High blood glucose, blood pressure and cholesterol can damage nerves so that they cannot send messages at all—or cannot send them correctly. This damage can occur in many parts of the body, including the intestines, heart and sex organs.

Neuropathy is another name for nerve damage.

You are less likely to have nerve damage (called **neuropathy**) if you can control your diabetes.

Two types of nerve damage are common in people with diabetes: **peripheral neuropathy** and **autonomic neuropathy.**

What is peripheral neuropathy?

Peripheral neuropathy is damage to the nerves in the muscles, legs and arms. Symptoms include:

Peripheral neuropathy is the most common type of nerve damage seen in people with diabetes.

- "pins and needles," tingling, numbness or burning in your hands, arms, legs or feet. The feelings are most common at night.

- loss of balance or coordination.

- feeling less sensitive to pain, heat or cold.

- sharp pains or cramps.

- feeling very sensitive to even a light touch.

Your doctor may prescribe pain medicine or other medicine to treat peripheral nerve damage.

What is autonomic neuropathy?

Autonomic neuropathy is damage to the nerves that control the bladder, stomach, intestines, sex organs, heart and blood pressure. It can cause the following problems:

Feeling dizzy or faint when changing positions (called *orthostatic hypotension*)

- **What is it?** Your blood pressure can drop suddenly as you stand, sit or lie down. You feel dizzy or as if you are going to faint.

- **How is it treated?** Do not stand, sit or lie down too quickly. Wear supportive (elastic) stockings. Raise the head of your bed. If prescribed by a doctor, take medicine to help keep sodium (salt) in your body.

Change in bowel (toilet) habits

- **What is it?** You may be constipated (have hard stools) or have diarrhea (loose stools) when you use the toilet.

- **How is it treated?** Take a laxative (to soften your stools) or anti-diarrhea medicine (to harden your stools). You can buy these at the drug store. Talk to your dietitian about how to adjust your diet.

Digestive problems (called *gastroparesis*)

- **What is it?** Food does not pass through your stomach as fast as usual. You may feel full or sick to your stomach. You may throw up. Your blood glucose will be harder to control because the food you eat is not digested normally.

- **How is it treated?** Eat smaller meals and eat more often. Decrease the fat and fiber in your diet. Talk to your dietitian about which foods you can eat to keep your blood glucose under good control. If prescribed by a doctor, take medicine to help food digest more quickly.

If you have digestive problems, it may be harder to control your blood glucose. See your doctor.

Sexual dysfunction (sexual response problems)

- **What is it?** If you are a man, you may have trouble getting or keeping an erection. If you are a woman, you may find it hard to become aroused or have an orgasm.

- **How is it treated?** See your doctor. If you are a man, ask about devices, medicines and other ways to help you get an erection. If you are a woman, ask about lubricants and help with arousal and orgasm problems. In either case, if you are using tobacco products, stop. And if you use alcohol heavily, cut back. See a counselor or therapist if sexual dysfunction becomes a major problem in your life.

Your doctor may refer you to a specialist, such as a urologist or gynecologist.

Problems emptying your bladder
(called *neurogenic bladder*)

- **What is it?** You have trouble emptying your bladder. This happens because the nerves that tell you when your bladder is full have been damaged.

- **How is it treated?** Try to urinate at regular times (every 3 hours, for example). If prescribed by a doctor, take medicine to help you empty your bladder. Your doctor may use a catheter (a tube put into the bladder to drain it) to empty your bladder. In some cases, surgery may be an option.

Being unaware when your blood glucose is low
(called *hypoglycemic unawareness*)

- **What is it?** You may no longer be able to tell when you have hypoglycemia (low blood glucose). This can be dangerous, especially if you drive or operate heavy equipment.

If you cannot tell when your blood glucose is low, you may need to check your glucose levels more often.

- **How is it treated?** You should work closely with your doctor to set a blood glucose range that is safe for you. It is very important that you check your blood glucose often, especially before you drive.

"Silent" heart attack

- **What is it?** Over time, damage to the nerves of the heart can lead to a heart attack with few or no symptoms. Women are at greater risk for "silent" heart attacks than men.

- **How is it treated?** If you have any sign of a problem or change in how you feel, seek medical care.

What can I do to prevent nerve damage?

- Keep your blood glucose in your target range. This can lower your risk of nerve disease up to 60 percent.

- Keep your blood pressure in your target range.

- Keep your cholesterol and triglycerides (blood fats) in your target range.

- If you smoke, ask your care provider for help with quitting.

- Check your feet every day for sores, redness or swelling. Wear well-fitting, supportive shoes.

- Limit your use of alcohol.

You may prevent nerve damage by controlling your blood glucose, blood pressure and cholesterol.

Taking care of your eyes

You will need to take good care of your eyes to prevent retinopathy, glaucoma and cataracts.

Your eyes have many small blood vessels that can be easily damaged by diabetes. A common problem for people with diabetes is a disease called **retinopathy.**

What is retinopathy?

Retinopathy is an eye disease that happens when tiny blood vessels in the eye become damaged and plugged. This causes other blood vessels in the eye to widen and leak, and new blood vessels begin to form. The new blood vessels are weak and bleed easily, which can affect your ability to see.

Having high blood glucose and high blood pressure over a long period of time increases your risk of retinopathy.

Are there other eye problems I should be concerned about?

Yes. Both glaucoma and cataracts are more common in people who have diabetes.

Glaucoma is increased pressure in the eye. Often there are no symptoms. Tell your doctor if you feel any pain in your eyes or if your vision changes.

Cataracts block or change the direction of light rays as they pass through the lens of your eye. They are more common—and appear at a younger age—in people with diabetes. Tell your doctor if you have any blurred vision or glare.

What can I do to protect my eyes and my vision?

To lower your risk of these eye problems:

- Have a yearly eye exam. Have your vision checked and your eyes examined and dilated at least once a year by an eye doctor (ophthalmologist).

- See an eye doctor at once if you notice any change in your eyes or vision.

- Control your blood glucose. Monitor your blood glucose regularly. Tell someone on your diabetes care team if your glucose levels change or you are having trouble staying in your target range.

- Keep your blood pressure below 130/80. Have your blood pressure checked every time you visit your doctor or clinic. If your blood pressure is too high, you may need to take medicine to lower it. Be sure to take your medicine regularly and in the way that your doctor has told you to take it.

It's important to have a yearly exam with an eye doctor (ophthalmologist).

Wear sunglasses that offer UVA or UVB protection.

- Protect your eyes by wearing glasses or other protective lenses as needed. Sunglasses with ultraviolet ray (UVA, UVB) protection will help protect your eyes from the sun.

- If you have signs of retinopathy, your eye doctor may suggest laser treatment. Laser treatment uses a light beam to seal off leaking blood vessels in the eye.

Diabetes and Eye Disease

Four out of five people with diabetes that has not been well controlled for at least 15 years have retinopathy. Many people have no symptoms until their vision begins to fail.

Diabetes is the leading cause of new cases of blindness in people between the ages of 24 and 70.

People with diabetes are 25 times more likely to become blind than those without diabetes.

Taking care of your feet

It is important to take good care of your feet so that small problems do not turn into big problems. High blood glucose can cause nerve disease, blood vessel disease and infections in the feet. With good diabetes control, foot problems can be prevented.

If you control your diabetes well, you should not have foot problems.

Nerve disease in the feet

High blood glucose can damage the nerves that send messages from your brain to your feet and back. When these nerves are damaged, you may not feel pain, heat or cold in your legs and feet. If you have sores or cuts on your feet, you may not know it. Small sores or cuts can lead to large sores and infections if not treated.

If you have nerve disease in your legs or feet, you may also have:

- numbness

- tingling

- burning

- pain

- balance problems.

Nerve damage can also weaken the muscles in the feet and shorten the tendons, changing the shape of your foot and how you walk.

Blood vessel disease in the legs and feet

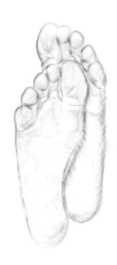

Healthy blood vessels keep your feet warm, heal wounds and fight infection. High blood glucose can damage the vessels so that your legs and feet do not get enough blood. This is called **peripheral artery disease.** Some symptoms include:

- pain when resting or sleeping

- pain in your calves when walking or running

- wounds that heal slowly or not at all

- coldness.

Infections in the feet

The job of white blood cells is to fight infection. But white blood cells cannot do this job well when blood glucose levels are high. As a result, wounds take longer to heal and small infections can become big problems.

Poor blood flow to the legs and feet can also cause wounds to heal more slowly. For these reasons, it is important to control your blood glucose.

How can I take good care of my feet?

- Control your blood glucose levels.

- Control your blood pressure.

- Control your cholesterol and triglycerides (blood fats).

- Avoid smoking and using tobacco.

- Check your feet every day for:

  - changes in color (from pink to white or blue), hair loss on the feet or toes, and unusual coldness.

  - signs of infection.

  - thick toenails, cracks or ridges, or fungus under the toenails.

  - blisters or corns.

  - cuts, drainage, cracking, peeling or any irritation of the skin.

  If you have problems seeing or reaching your feet, ask your diabetes care team about getting a mirror with a long handle. This will allow you to see the bottom of your feet.

- Keep your feet clean and dry. Do not soak your feet. You can put creams on your feet and legs, but not between your toes.

Check your feet each day for wounds that are healing too slowly. Report any problems to your doctor.

A long-handled mirror can help you see the bottom of your feet.

- Trim your toenails in the shape of your toes. The best time to trim your nails is after a shower or bath when your nails are soft and will not splinter or crack. See a foot doctor (podiatrist) if your nails are very thick or break easily, you have foot problems that need attention, or you cannot take care of your nails by yourself.

- Do not go barefoot. You may injure your foot on something sharp without knowing it.

- Wear good footwear. Make sure your shoes fit well and your toes have enough room.

- Check the inside of your shoe to make sure there are no rough or thick seams. The sole of the shoe should be firm for safe walking. Always fit new shoes to both feet, because they may not be the same size and shape. Shop for shoes at the end of the day when your feet may be somewhat larger. Replace your shoes regularly.

- Wear polyester socks that take moisture away from the feet. They should not have any seams, creases or elastic that would press on your feet. Change your socks regularly to keep your feet clean and dry.

It's a good idea to shop for shoes at the end of the day, when your feet are a little larger.

- Do not use hot water bottles or heating pads. Do not treat foot problems yourself with non-prescription (over-the-counter) remedies.

- Always check the temperature of water on the inside of your wrist before washing yourself or stepping into a bathtub.

- Have your feet checked every time you see your doctor. Take your shoes and socks off so your doctor is sure to look at them. Call your doctor if you see signs of infection or other problems with your feet.

Ask your doctor to check for peripheral artery disease.

- Ask your doctor to check the nerves in your feet using a **monofilament.** This is like a hairbrush with a single bristle. Your doctor will press it gently against the bottoms of your feet to see what you can feel.

- Your doctor will check how well blood is flowing to your legs and feet by checking the pulses in your feet.

Taking care of your teeth and gums

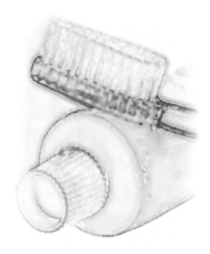

Diabetes that is not well controlled can affect the health of your teeth and gums.

Plaque build-up on teeth is a breeding ground for germs. High blood glucose raises the risk of mouth infections because germs feed on glucose. And infection raises your blood glucose even higher.

To care for your teeth and gums:

- Brush with a soft toothbrush and floss your teeth regularly.

It is important to take good care of your teeth and gums. This helps prevent tooth decay and mouth infections.

- Visit your dentist every six months for an exam and cleaning. Make sure your dentist knows that you have diabetes.

- If you wear dentures, keep them very clean, brushing them daily.

- See a dentist as soon as you can if you notice any changes in your teeth or gums, especially signs of an infection, or if you have any problems that do not go away. Red, sore and bleeding gums are the first signs of gum disease.

- Change your toothbrush regularly.

- Control your blood glucose.

- Eat a healthy diet.

- Do not smoke or use tobacco.

Preventing infection and injury

It is important for people with diabetes to try to avoid infection and injury.

Having an infection causes blood glucose to rise. High blood glucose can also make it easier for you to get an infection. Good glucose control can prevent infections.

To prevent infections and injuries:

- Keep your skin clean and dry. If your skin is too dry, use skin lotion or cream.

- Eat a healthy diet.

- Do not smoke or use tobacco.

- Control your blood glucose.

- Treat cuts, broken skin or burns quickly. Keep injuries clean and watch for any signs of infection. Call your doctor if you think you may have an infection or if you have problems that do not go away.

- Be careful when you shave. Use an electric razor, if you can, so that you are less likely to cut yourself.

Some Signs of Infection

Warmth, redness, tenderness or swelling

Pain or a burning feeling

Fever

Pus or drainage

A tired or sick feeling

You will want to do everything you can to avoid infections. Infections will cause your blood glucose to rise—and high blood glucose may lead to more infections.

- Protect your skin, including your feet, from the sun. Wear sunscreen and appropriate clothing and shoes.

- To keep your blood flowing:
  - do not wear stockings or hose that are too tight.
  - try not to cross your legs while sitting.
  - raise your feet if they become swollen, then call your doctor.

- Prevent bladder infections by drinking plenty of water.

Make sure you are up to date on all your shots, including for flu, pneumonia and tetanus.

- Get a flu vaccine once a year.

- Get a pneumococcal (pneumonia) vaccine every 5 years.

- Get a tetanus vaccine every 10 years.

- Get other vaccinations as appropriate. (Talk with your doctor for more information.)

Chapter 8

Day-to-Day Living

➤ Changes in your daily routine can cause blood glucose levels to rise or fall. Since no one has the exact same routine each day, it helps to know how to head off problems before they occur.

➤ Be smart about alcohol, tobacco, medicines and other drugs. Learn how these affect your blood glucose levels.

➤ When you are sick, your blood glucose levels will rise. You can follow simple steps to help manage diabetes on sick days.

➤ You *can* travel safely with diabetes. The key is knowing how to prepare. You will find a packing list and guidelines later in this chapter. Your diabetes care team will tell you if your treatment plan needs to change while you're away from home.

➤ Never drive if your blood glucose is below 100. Keep juice, crackers or other carbohydrates in the car in case of delays.

As you get used to managing your diabetes, it will become a "normal" part of your life. You will know what to do if your blood glucose level goes down, what to eat throughout the day and how to take good care of yourself to prevent problems.

Yet each day brings new challenges. You may wonder if you can drink at a party, or how to take care of yourself on sick days. You may not know what to pack for vacation. You might worry about your blood glucose dropping if you are delayed in traffic.

This section describes common concerns and tips for dealing with the unexpected.

What should I know about alcohol, tobacco, medicines and other drugs?

Alcohol

Drinking alcohol can:

If you choose to drink alcohol, be sensible. Drink in moderation.

- make you gain weight.

- worsen diseases related to diabetes.

- make you less alert.

- affect your ability to drive safely.

- interact in bad ways with the medicines you take.

Alcohol's effect on your blood glucose will vary. It will depend on what you drink, how much you drink and whether you have eaten any food.

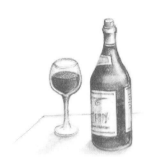

- Alcohol can keep your liver from releasing glucose. (Normally, your liver releases glucose when you have not eaten for a while. This keeps your blood glucose from falling too low.)

- If you drink without eating food, you can get hypoglycemia (low blood glucose). This is especially true if you take insulin, sulfonylureas or meglitinides. (See Know Your Medicines, chapter 4.)

- If you have been drinking, you and others around you may not know if your glucose level drops. Some of the effects of alcohol are similar to the symptoms of low blood glucose—for example, dizziness or weakness.

- Alcohol can raise your blood glucose if you drink sugary drinks or mixers that contain sugar, or if you drink too much at one time.

If you choose to drink alcohol:

- **Check your blood glucose often while you are drinking** to see how the alcohol is affecting you. Always check your blood glucose before you go to bed after you have been drinking, especially if you have

Alcohol can lower your blood glucose for up to 12 hours after you drink.

also been physically active. Dancing, sports and other physical activity will increase your risk of hypoglycemia (low blood glucose) later on.

- **Eat food while drinking alcohol,** especially food that contains carbohydrate. This may help you avoid low blood glucose.

- **Limit the amount of alcohol that you drink.** If you are a woman, drink no more than one serving of alcohol a day. If you are a man, drink no more than two servings of alcohol a day. A serving of alcohol equals:

    - 12 ounces of beer.

    - 5 ounces of wine.

    - 1½ ounces of liquor.

- **Be aware of how drinks with soda, juice, milk or cream can affect you.** Such "mixes" may contain calories or carbohydrates that can raise your blood glucose. Examples include piña coladas, rum and Cokes, margaritas and daiquiris. Use such drinks with moderation. Be sure to count high-carbohydrate mixers in your meal plan. When possible, try to use diet soda, club soda or water rather than high-carbohydrate mixers.

Mixers often contain calories and carbohydrates.

- **Wear medical identification (ID) that says you have diabetes.**

- Use alcohol only when your blood glucose is under control.

- **Know that you may have hypoglycemia (low blood glucose) if you drink alcohol while taking medicine that lowers blood glucose.** Your skin may become flushed, you may feel sick to your stomach, your heart may beat fast or you may have trouble speaking.

- **If you take metformin (Glucophage), you should not use alcohol without first talking with your doctor.**

- **If you have a history of abusing alcohol, you should not use alcohol.**

- **If you are pregnant, you should not use alcohol.**

- **If you have certain diseases, you should cut back on or stop using alcohol.** These include pancreatitis (inflammation of the pancreas), dyslipidemia (high levels of fat in the blood) or neuropathy (nerve disease).

Almost one out of three people who use hypoglycemic medicine have a reaction when they drink alcohol.

Tobacco

Smoking—or inhaling someone else's smoke—greatly increases your risk for serious disease.

Both smoking (cigarettes, cigars or pipes) and using smokeless tobacco (chewing tobacco or snuff) will harm your body, especially if you have diabetes. Smoking increases your risk of heart, kidney, nerve and eye disease.

When you smoke, chew or inhale tobacco, nicotine enters your bloodstream. This causes your blood vessels to narrow, reducing blood flow to all parts of your body. Even secondhand smoke is harmful to your health and should be avoided.

People who use smokeless tobacco are two to three times more likely to have gum disease and other severe dental problems than people who do not use smokeless tobacco.

Smokeless tobacco can cause white, leathery patches to form on the inside of your cheek or gum. These white patches can develop into cancer of the mouth, involving the lip, tongue or cheek.

If you want to lower your risk of problems from diabetes, you should **quit using tobacco.** Tell your doctor that you want to take advantage of the many resources to help you quit, including:

- local support groups

- the American Lung Association

- Internet resources

- the toll-free state tobacco help line (1-877-270-STOP).

Support, counseling and medicines (like nicotine patches or gum) are all helpful in quitting tobacco.

Illegal drugs

Illegal drugs can keep you from making good decisions about your diabetes. They can also threaten your physical and emotional health. When you use illegal drugs, you are less likely to:

Examples of illegal drugs include marijuana, methamphetamine, heroin and cocaine.

- exercise and eat well

- recognize and treat the signs of high or low blood glucose

- drive safely

- cooperate with others to live well and manage your diabetes.

Your risk of heart attack and stroke goes up when you use illegal drugs. If you are pregnant, the risk that your fetus will be harmed also increases. Tell your doctor if you are using any illegal drugs, and seek help to stop using them.

Medicines

If you take any prescription or non-prescription medicines, it is important that you know:

- the name of the medicine and what it is for

- what it does

- what the possible side effects are

- how to take it safely.

Your Medicine List

Keep an updated list of all your medicines, herbal products and vitamin and mineral supplements. Have this with you at all times for clinic visits and in case of emergencies.

If you are allergic to any medicines, write this on your list as well. If your allergy is life-threatening, you should wear a bracelet or necklace that says this.

Herbal products and vitamin tablets can affect your medicines. Tell your doctor about any supplements you take.

If you are taking more than one medicine, you also need to know how they may interact with each other. The best source of this information is your doctor or pharmacist.

Use the following guide before taking any over-the-counter medicine. Ask your care provider or pharmacist which product is best for you. Remember to test your blood glucose levels to see how the medicine affects your blood glucose.

What can I take for aches, pains, fever and inflammation?

Tylenol (acetaminophen) is best. It will not affect your blood glucose and will not harm your kidneys. Do not use this if you have liver disease.

Aspirin is usually safe for most people. Note that large doses (more than 8 tablets a day) can cause your blood glucose to drop (hypoglycemia).

Check with your doctor before using Advil (ibuprofen), Aleve (naprosyn), Orudis KT or Actron (ketoprofen), or other drugs. These may cause your blood pressure to rise. They may also affect your kidneys.

If you have high blood pressure or kidney disease, you should avoid non-steroidal anti-inflammatory medicines.

What can I take for a runny nose, itchy or watery eyes and sneezing?

Antihistamines are best. These include Claritin (loratadine), Benadryl (diphenhydramine) and Chlor-Trimeton (chlorpheniramine).

Note: These drugs may cause dry mouth and constipation (hard dry stools that are difficult to pass). Most can make you tired or drowsy. (Claritin should not make you drowsy). Confusion may occur in elderly people.

Avoid eye drops that contain a decongestant. These can increase blood pressure.

If you have narrow-angle glaucoma, you should avoid Visine, Naphcon-A and other eye drops. These can increase the pressure in your eyes.

What can I take for a stuffy nose or congested (plugged-up) sinuses?

Try a **nasal spray** like Afrin (oxymetazoline). Use caution with nasal sprays. Do not use them for more than 3 to 5 days in a row, or they might make your congestion worse.

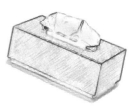

Do not use Sudafed (pseudoephedrine) or other oral decongestants. These may cause your blood pressure to go up.

To help with a dry, irritated nose, try a saline spray such as Ocean Mist.

What can I use for a cough or scratchy throat?

Cough drops, sugar-free candy or **sugar-free gum** may help a scratchy throat.

Expectorants (guaifenesin) will help a productive cough. Large amounts of water will also help clear the mucus from your lungs.

A **cough suppressant (dextromethorphan)** may help a dry cough. Do not use this with a productive or congested cough.

Use a cough suppressant for a dry cough. Use an expectorant for a productive cough.

If you take cough syrup, check the ingredients on the label. If it contains sugar, it may affect your blood glucose levels. You may want to keep track of the carbohydrates.

What can I do for an upset stomach or heartburn?

Antacids (Maalox, Mylanta, TUMS) work well, but they may cause diarrhea (loose, watery stools) or constipation (hard, dry stools). Watch the sugar content in TUMS if you use it often.

Avoid Tagamet HB. This interacts with many drugs, including diabetes medicines. Pepcid AC, Axid AR, Zantac 75 and Prilosec OTC are often safer.

Can I use diet aids?

Try to avoid diet aids. Many contain stimulants. They may raise your blood pressure and blood glucose, and they could increase the risk of stroke.

What can I do for constipation?

Before trying any medicine, **increase your fluids (especially water), fiber and exercise.** See chapter 5 for the fiber content in common foods.

If you choose to use a laxative, don't use it for more than one week. If constipation lasts more than a week, call your doctor.

- You may want to try bulk-forming laxatives such as **sugar-free Citrucel, Fibercon or Metamucil.**

- Do not use stimulant laxatives such as bisacodyl (Dulcolax) or senna (Senokot).

- To prevent constipation, you may try emollient laxatives such as docusate (Colace). These are stool softeners.

More fluids, fiber and exercise are the first choice in treating constipation.

What can I do for diarrhea?

Do not treat diarrhea yourself. Call your doctor.

Diarrhea can cause dehydration (a loss of fluids in the body). It is best to call your doctor before treating diarrhea yourself.

What should I take if I cannot sleep?

You might try **diphenhydramine (Sominex, Benadryl, Unisom)** or **doxylamine (Unisom Nighttime Sleep Aid)**. These are antihistamines. Side effects include dry mouth and constipation (hard dry stools that are difficult to pass). Confusion may occur in elderly people.

Avoid products that contain aspirin or magnesium salicylate (such as Alka-Seltzer PM, Bayer PM and Doans PM).

Dietary Supplements

Dietary supplements include vitamins, minerals, nutrition drinks and other products that add nutrients to your body. These products may affect your blood glucose. You will need to test your glucose levels when stopping or starting a supplement.

Talk to your care team before taking any supplements. Everyone reacts to these products differently. Ask yourself:

1. How will this product affect my glucose control? Will it lower or increase my glucose?

2. Is this product safe for me to take? What are the side effects? Does it interact with any of my other medicines?

3. How much should I take? How often should I take it?

4. What product or brand is best for me?

As with any medicine, you should think carefully before taking a dietary supplement.

The companies that make supplements are not required to prove their safety and effectiveness to the Food and Drug Administration. Products vary in quality and strength. If you have questions about a product or brand, talk to your pharmacist.

How should I handle sick days?

Illness can cause your blood glucose to rise.

You may need to test your blood glucose more often on days that you are sick.

When you are sick, your blood glucose may be higher than usual. Being sick stresses the body, and stress can cause your blood glucose to rise.

If you are sick, it is important to do the following:

- **Always take your diabetes medicine or insulin, even if you can't eat.** Ask your diabetes care team if you should change the amount of medicine or insulin you take when you are sick.

- **Test your blood glucose often:** before every meal and at bedtime or every 4 hours during the day. Record your blood glucose levels in your record book or journal.

- **Drink at least 1 cup (8 ounces) of caffeine-free, calorie-free liquid every hour while awake.** This will help keep you from getting dehydrated (losing too many fluids). Some options include:

  Water

  Tea (no caffeine)

  Clear broth

  Diet soda pop

- **If your stomach is upset and you cannot eat your regular foods:** eat or drink 15 grams of carbohydrate (or other easy-to-digest solid food) every hour while awake.

This is in addition to liquids every hour. Some options include:

  ½ cup fruit juice

  ½ cup regular (not diet) soda pop

  1 Popsicle

  ½ cup regular Jell-O

  5 to 6 saltine crackers

  1 piece dry toast.

If you live alone, always keep some sick-day foods handy in case you are unable to go to the store to buy them.

Call your doctor if:

- your blood glucose has been over 240 for longer than a day.

- you are throwing up for more than 6 hours.

- you have diarrhea (loose stools) for more than 6 hours.

- you feel sleepier than usual.

- you have trouble breathing.

- you are unable to think clearly.

If you have to go to the hospital, ask to see a diabetes doctor (endocrinologist).

If You Go to the Hospital

Bring your blood glucose meter with you.

Have your blood glucose checked every 4 hours. If your blood glucose level is over 180, you should get treatment to lower it.

Ask for an endocrinologist (diabetes doctor) to be on your hospital care team.

Share this information with family, friends or others who might be asked to help make decisions for you, in case you are unable to make them yourself.

How can I get ready for travel?

Traveling with diabetes involves some planning ahead. Here are a few tips:

- **See your doctor well before leaving the country to get any shots you will need.** You may need immunizations if you will travel abroad or be gone for a while.

- **Before you leave, see your doctor to get any prescriptions you might need.** Ask your doctor to sign a letter explaining your treatment plan and medicines. You may need prescriptions for one or more of the following:

- insulin
- oral medicines
- glucagon kit
- blood glucose meter and testing supplies
- insulin pump and supplies
- medicines for nausea and vomiting.

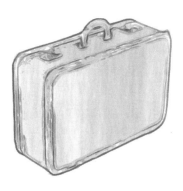

- **Ask your diabetes care team:**
  - how to adjust your schedule for taking insulin and medicines when you cross a time zone
  - whether you will need nausea or diarrhea medicines or prescriptions
  - whether you will need a glucagon kit or prescription.

- **Pack your blood glucose testing supplies, insulin and insulin supplies, medicines and food that you will need for your trip.** You should have an extra week's worth of supplies in case something is lost or damaged.

- **Make sure the people you are traveling with know about your diabetes and treatment plan.**

- **Find out how and where to get medical care where you will be traveling.**

Do not expect to buy extra supplies when you are traveling, especially if you are going to another country. Different countries use different kinds of insulin, needles and pills.

What should I keep with me during travel?

Carry all of your diabetes supplies with you, especially your medicines. Never pack your supplies in your checked bags.

Never pack your insulin in your checked baggage.

If you can, set aside at least a couple of extra days of diabetes supplies (except insulin) in a separate place—in a handbag or with someone traveling with you—just in case the supplies you carry are lost or stolen.

Besides your diabetes supplies:

- Always carry some form of carbohydrate to treat hypoglycemia (low blood glucose).

- Carry some food and snacks in case a flight is cancelled, meals are delayed or places that sell food are closed.

- Make sure you have your doctor's name, phone number and fax number in case you or someone else has to reach him or her. Also, be sure to carry your own address and phone number, your medical insurance card, and an emergency name, address and phone number.

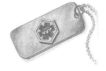

- Make sure you have a medical identification (ID) bracelet or necklace and a wallet card with you at all times.

Packing List for Travelers

❏ Prescriptions for insulin, medicines and other supplies

❏ Blood glucose testing supplies

❏ Insulin and insulin supplies

❏ Medicines

❏ Foods with carbohydrate

❏ Phone numbers for local clinics and hospitals that can provide medical care, if you need it while traveling

❏ Your doctor's name, phone number and fax number

❏ Your own address and phone number, as well as an emergency name, address and phone number

❏ Medical ID (wallet card and bracelet or necklace)

❏ Your medical insurance card

❏ Two pairs of shoes, plus sandals or other swim shoes

❏ Sunglasses and sunscreen

Try to bring an extra week's worth of diabetes supplies. Pack supplies in your carry-on bag. Set aside a few days' worth in another place (with a fellow traveler, for example), in case your carry-on bag is lost or stolen.

Can I take needles, lancets and medicines on an airplane?

Yes. But you will need to do the following.

- **Keep your insulin and other medicines in their original packages with printed prescription labels on each.** This is required by the Federal Aviation Administration. As long as your insulin is in its original package with your name and prescription number, taking syringes on board will not be a problem.

You can take needles on a plane as long as your insulin is in its original package with your name and prescription number.

- **Make sure your glucose meter has the brand name on it.** This is needed for you to take lancets or needles on board the plane.

How can I manage my diabetes away from home?

- **Protect your feet.** Wear shoes that fit well, and take at least two pairs of shoes with you. Make sure your shoes have been broken in and are comfortable, as you will most likely be walking a lot on your trip. Bring sandals, flip-flops or swim shoes for the beach, as well as for your hotel room.

- **Protect your eyes with sunglasses.**

- **Protect your skin from sunburn.** Bring sunscreen, and wear it. Remember that the tops of your feet and head can burn, too.

- **Plan to rest and exercise properly during your trip.** However you travel, stretch and walk around every one to two hours.

- **Be ready to treat low blood glucose if you exercise more than usual on your trip.** Carry a carbohydrate with you at all times, and tell a travel partner how to help in case of an emergency. You may need to eat more food or use less insulin (if you take insulin) if you are more active than usual.

Make sure your fellow travelers know you have diabetes—and how to help you in an emergency.

- **Check your blood glucose often during your trip.** Because you are eating new foods, doing new things and changing your routine, you will need to monitor your blood glucose more than usual. Protect your testing supplies and carry prescriptions for them in case they are lost or damaged. Throw away any used needles and lancets in a safe manner.

Always throw needles and lancets away in a safe manner.

What about insulin?

If you take insulin and you know that you are going to cross a time zone during your trip, talk with your diabetes care team at least two weeks before you leave. Ask them how to adjust your treatment plan.

You may need to take more or less insulin when you change time zones. Ask your diabetes care team.

In general: When you travel east, you lose hours from your day, so you may need less insulin. When you travel west, you add hours to your day, so you may need more insulin. This will vary depending on the type of insulin you take.

If you wear an insulin pump, it is important to change the times for your basal rate when you reach your destination. You will need to change how you take your insulin as your meal times, sleep times and blood glucose levels change.

How do I know when it's safe for me to drive?

When your blood glucose is too low, it can affect your judgment. And when your judgment is affected, your ability to drive is also affected. Hypoglycemia (low blood glucose) is especially a problem when you are driving.

Your blood glucose should be at least 100 before you drive.

To drive more safely:

- **Plan all trips carefully so as to not miss meals or snacks.**

- **Check your blood glucose before you drive.** If it is below 70, eat 15 grams of carbohydrate, then check it again 15 minutes later. Your blood glucose should be at least 100 before you drive.

- **Keep blood glucose testing equipment with you in your car.**

- **Keep some form of carbohydrate in your car at all times.** For example: fruit, crackers or small juice boxes.

- **If you are unable to check your blood glucose, and two hours have gone by since you last ate, eat 15 grams of carbohydrate before driving.**

Traffic delays and accidents make driving time hard to predict. Always keep carbohydrates in your car, just in case.

- **Check your blood glucose every two hours during a trip.** Treat hypoglycemia (low blood glucose) by pulling to the side of the road and eating or drinking 15 grams of carbohydrate. Wait 20 to 30 minutes to make sure that your blood glucose is in a safe range before you drive again. Do not drive until your symptoms are gone and your blood glucose is over 100.

- **Do not drive after drinking alcohol.** Alcohol lowers your blood glucose and may keep you from driving safely.

Chapter 9

Accepting Your Diagnosis

➤ It's true that diabetes will change your life. You will likely move through several stages of loss before you can accept that you have this disease. This is normal.

➤ Coping with diabetes can be stressful. But remember that stress can raise your blood glucose levels. It's important to learn healthy ways to cope with stress.

➤ Depression is common in people who have diabetes. If you are depressed for more than two weeks, you need to get help.

➤ You will need all the support you can get as you adjust to your new life with diabetes. Tell family and friends what you need. Think about joining a diabetes support group.

When you were told you have diabetes, you suffered a kind of loss. You may feel you've lost the body you had, your health, or your sense of independence.

This loss will take time to accept. But you *can* adjust to it—and live a full, enjoyable, healthy life with diabetes. It will take some time and often some work.

Adjusting to your loss

People often adjust to loss in stages that include denial, bargaining, anger, sadness and acceptance.

Denial

It's normal to want to deny you have diabetes at first. Many people do. It takes time to get used to the idea.

Often, the first thing people feel when they learn they have diabetes is denial: "This can't be happening to me. There must be some mistake. The lab results must be wrong."

This is a very common response. If you are feeling this way you are not alone. It will take time to get used to the idea that diabetes is now part of your life. Denial can keep you from recognizing the need to take care of your diabetes.

Bargaining

Bargaining often follows denial. You may think, "If I am really good, this will get better and go away." Unfortunately, diabetes does not go away.

Often, people newly diagnosed with diabetes work hard and do very well for the first six months or so after diagnosis. Then they begin to forget to do the things they need to do to control their diabetes. When this happens, the diabetes may become harder to control.

It is not easy to see diabetes as a lifetime issue that requires ongoing care.

Anger

You did not deserve to get diabetes. No matter how much you weigh or how active you are, there is someone who weighs more and exercises less but does not have diabetes. We know diabetes is caused in part by the genes you inherited from your parents. It is not your fault you got those genes. Diabetes is one of those bad things that just happens sometimes.

Anger is a reasonable reaction when bad things happen in life.

Some people will turn the anger on themselves, telling themselves that if they had been doing things differently they would not now have diabetes. No one can tell you whether this is true or not. And feeling guilty is not going to help things get better.

If you are angry, you may be irritable and more easily annoyed. Try to release your anger in ways that will not harm your relationships. Physical activity and talking with others may help to relieve your feelings.

If you are feeling guilty about getting diabetes, talk about it with someone. You need to believe that you are not to blame for this happening.

Diabetes does not have to cause bad things to happen. Fear, anger and sadness does not need to rule your life.

Sadness

You may feel a strong sense of sadness when you learn you have diabetes. You may feel overwhelmed and unable to cope with the things you must do to manage diabetes. You may even feel that your life is less fulfilling or valuable now.

It is important to talk with someone about these feelings and begin to work your way through them.

Acceptance

Now that you are diagnosed with diabetes, the real question is, what are you going to do about it?

You need to work through the stages of denial, bargaining, anger and sadness to get to the point of acceptance. Once you accept that you have diabetes, that it's not going away and that there is no one to blame (not even yourself), it will be easier to do what you need to do to be healthy.

How do I deal with these feelings?

These feelings are normal and can occur in any order. They may even return when something bad happens, whether or not it's connected to your diabetes. For example, a death, illness or crisis all can trigger old feelings of anger or sadness.

Be aware of your feelings. Know that getting "stuck" in any stage for too long can lead to poor self-care. It can also disrupt your relationships and daily activities.

Discuss your feelings with your care team, and talk to loved ones who will listen and understand. This will help you move on, feel better and take better care of your diabetes and yourself.

Managing stress

Stress, whether positive or negative, can cause your blood glucose to rise. When you are stressed, your liver releases glucose into the bloodstream. This gives you energy to deal with whatever is causing your stress. (It is sometimes called the "fight or flight" response.)

If you have diabetes, being stressed may cause your liver to release too much glucose. So, to manage your diabetes, you have to learn to manage your stress.

Some kinds of stress are hard to avoid, like the stress of being in a car accident or losing a job. But people can make stress better or worse by the kinds of messages they tell themselves.

If you tell yourself that losing a job is an opportunity to find another, better job, you are causing yourself less stress than if you tell yourself that you will never find another job and will soon be homeless. Check out the messages that you are giving yourself.

You can lessen your stress by breathing deeply, meditating or praying, and exercising. Focus your mind on the present moment, notice what is around you and find what there is to enjoy in that moment. Remember, most of what we worry about is in the past or in the future. But we are only alive in the present.

Sometimes there may be ongoing stressful situations that can make your diabetes harder to control. These situations often can be improved by making some changes in your life.

- First you need to recognize what is causing your stress. You may have to look carefully at your life to see what is contributing to your stress.

- Next, look at what part of the situation is beyond your control and what part you could possibly change.

- Make plans to change the part you can change. Have a backup plan in case the first idea does not work out.

- Identify what is needed to make the plan work. What do you need to do? What are your strengths and where do you need help? Who can help you?

You can't avoid stress. But you can learn healthy ways to cope with it. This will help keep your blood glucose in a normal range.

Depression

Depression is more common in people with diabetes. At any given time, about one in three people with diabetes suffer from symptoms of depression. We do not know if this is because diabetes causes changes in the body that make depression more likely, or simply because diabetes can be stressful to live with.

When people are depressed, they do not take care of themselves as well as they normally do. This can make a big difference in diabetes care. If it is hard just to get out of bed in the morning, think how much harder it will be to monitor blood glucose, stay active and eat the right foods.

Remember that your diabetes care team is there to help. They understand the problems faced by people with diabetes.

Depression is a normal response to events that change our lives in ways that we do not like. But people who are depressed may need help from others to get better. Over time, physical changes can take place that can make depression harder to get over on your own.

How do I know if I am depressed?

The most common sign is that you no longer enjoy things you used to enjoy. There are other signs as well—not ever being hungry or eating all the time, being unable to sleep well or sleeping all the time, feeling sad or feeling irritable. Most people who are depressed feel that life has become bleak and gray.

What should I do if I think I'm depressed?

If you believe that you are depressed, talk with your family doctor. Tell your doctor how you feel. You may need medicine, counseling or both to help you get back to your normal self. It is up to you and your doctor to decide on a plan that works best for you.

If you have symptoms of depression for more than two weeks, it's time to get help. Call your doctor.

Are You Depressed?

1. Over the past two weeks, have you felt down, depressed or hopeless? ❑ yes ❑ no

2. Have you felt little interest or pleasure in the things you normally enjoy? ❑ yes ❑ no

If you answered yes to both questions, you may be depressed. It's important to call your care provider for help. Most people cannot treat depression by themselves.

Resources to Help with Depression

Depression and Bipolar Support Alliance: 800-826-3632, www.dbsalliance.org

National Institute of Mental Health: 800-421-4211, www.nimh.mh.gov

National Association of Cognitive-Behavioral Therapists: 800-853-1135, www.nacbt.org

National Mental Health Association: 800-969-0642, www.nmha.org

Fairview Mental Health Clinics:

Burnsville – 612-672-6999
Fairview Behavioral Services
156 Cobblestone Lane, Burnsville, MN 55337

Eden Prairie – 612-672-6999
Fairview Eden Center Clinic
830 Prairie Center Drive, Eden Prairie, MN 55344

Edina – 612-672-6999
Southdale Place
3400 W. 66th Street, Suite 400, Edina, MN 55435

Elk River – 763-241-5870

Fairview Northland Medical Building

290 Main Street, Suite 140, Elk River, MN 55330

Forest Lake– 612-672-6999

246 11th Avenue S.E., Forest Lake, MN 55025

Maplewood – 612-672-6999

2785 White Bear Avenue, Suite 108, Maplewood, MN 55109

Milaca – 320-983-7445

Fairview Milaca Health Care Center

150 10th Street NW, Milaca, MN 56363

Minneapolis – 612-672-6999

University of Minnesota Medical Center, Fairview
(formerly Fairview-University Medical Center)
Riverside West, Suite 1000, 2450 Riverside Avenue,
Minneapolis, MN 55454

Princeton – 763-389-6326

Fairview Northland Regional Medical Center

911 Northland Drive, Princeton, MN 55371

Zimmerman – 763-241-5870

Fairview Northland Zimmerman Clinic

25945 Gateway Drive, Zimmerman, MN 55398

Getting support

Finding out that you have diabetes puts demands not only on you but also on those close to you. The changes you must make to manage your diabetes can frustrate, confuse and even anger your family and friends.

Learning that you have diabetes affects how you feel about yourself, and this affects how you feel about those close to you.

Family and friends may go through stages of acceptance similar to what you are going through, although not always at the same time. Your loved ones may be afraid of possible complications, or how your treatment plan will affect their lives.

It is very important that you communicate with your family and friends. Involve them as you learn about diabetes and how to manage it. Their support will be a great help to you.

How can I get the support I need?

Your family and friends cannot help you unless you tell them that you need help.

When you ask for support, you should:

- **Say exactly what you need.** Don't make your family and friends have to guess what you mean. They may guess wrong.

- **Explain what you need in a positive way.** Ask for help. Do not complain about the lack of help. No one likes to be criticized.

- **Ask only for things that you know your family and friends can give you.** Do not ask for things they cannot do or are not yet ready to do. Be patient and help your family and friends learn with you.

- **Thank your family and friends when they give you the support you need.** This not only lets them know that they are helping you, but makes them want to do even more.

It's important to communicate your needs clearly and without criticism.

It's hard for people to understand what you're going through unless they have diabetes themselves. That's why support groups are so helpful.

No matter how much your family and friend may care about you and want to help you, they may not be able to give you all the support you need. This is why many people with diabetes join a diabetes support group.

Your health care team can help you locate a support group in your area. Or you can call one of the resources listed below for help.

- American Association of Diabetes Educators: 800-832-6874

- American Diabetes Association: 800-832-6874

- Juvenile Diabetes Research Foundation: 800-533-2873

- American Dietetic Association: 800-366-1655

Communicating with your care team

To manage your diabetes well, you need to become an active partner with your diabetes care team. The more active you are in your medical care, the better your care will be. After all, you are the one who lives with your diabetes every day.

You are the most important member of your care team.

Every member of your diabetes care team depends on you to share openly and honestly your concerns about your diabetes and how it is affecting you.

What can I do to be a good partner?

Know your disease. Learn, read, go to classes, ask questions. Replace fear with knowledge.

Know yourself. Be honest with yourself about how you feel about having diabetes, managing your diabetes and getting support.

Know your diabetes care team. Know who is on your team and how to contact them.

Know what you expect of your diabetes care team. Your care team should advise you, answer your questions and help you manage your diabetes well.

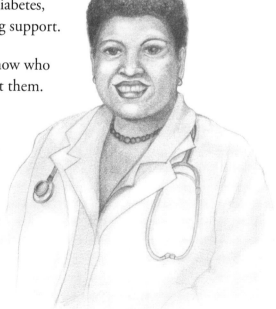

How can I prepare for visits with my care team?

To be a good partner, it helps to be prepared for each visit with your diabetes care team. Here are some tips for preparing for your regular visits:

- Collect the information you need for your visit. Have your glucose record book and your meter ready to take along. Bring a list of all the medicines that you take every day.

If you have taken your temperature, write it down and bring it with you to clinic visits.

- Write down any questions you may have so that you do not forget them.

- If things are happening to your body that you think may be because of your diabetes, write these things down. This will help you describe them better to your diabetes care team.

How can I get the most out of these visits?

Here are some things you can do to have a good visit with your diabetes care team.

- Tell your team if you have been feeling any stress.

- Be honest about your blood glucose readings and diabetes care. The more honest you are, the more helpful your diabetes care team can be.

- Wear short sleeves or a sleeveless top. This makes it easier to take your blood pressure.

- Wear about the same amount of clothing at each visit, so your weight can be compared with your weight at other visits.

Your blood pressure should be measured at each visit.

- Bring your glucose record book and your meter with you. Share the book with your care provider.

- Take off your shoes and socks so that your feet can be checked at every visit.

- Ask for an A1c test every 3 to 6 months.

- Ask for a urine test for protein at least once a year.

- Ask for a blood test for cholesterol and triglycerides (blood fats) at least once a year.

- When needed, ask for a referral to an eye doctor, foot doctor or other specialist. You should have an eye exam once a year.

Ask for brochures or other written materials that explain your medicines and instructions for care.

- Be sure you understand all the information that is given to you. Ask that the information be repeated and written down.

Track your test results so that you can see patterns in your blood glucose levels over time. You can use a notebook or diary, a foldout card or a computer file. Tracking your test results makes you a valuable partner in your diabetes care.

Chapter 10

Your Diabetes Care Plan

➤ There is a lot to learn about diabetes. It takes work, commitment and support to manage your blood glucose and be healthy.

➤ Diabetes will always be a part of your life. But if you manage it well, it doesn't have to run your life.

➤ To stay on track, it helps to set realistic goals for yourself. Make a plan you can stick to.

➤ You can use this chapter to keep track of your goals for blood glucose, exercise, meal planning, weight and other aspects of self-care.

Now that you know the basics, how do you go about living with diabetes day after day?

- **Keep learning.** Knowledge about diabetes grows and changes. Use your care team and other resources to stay up to date on diabetes care.

- **Keep connected.** You need people around you to help you manage your diabetes. This includes your family, friends and care team. Choose care providers you can work with, and see them regularly.

- **Keep positive.** Diabetes can be managed. It should be part of your life, not all of it. What you do matters. Your hard work will pay off.

- **Keep at it.** There will be times when things do not go as planned. This is normal. It is important to know when you are off track and how to get back on. You can learn a lot from the these times to help you do better in the future.

- **Keep focused.** The best way to stay on track is to stay organized. Set goals for yourself and take steps to reach them. Once you reach these goals, it is time to set new ones.

Setting goals

For goals to be useful, they should be:

- **Detailed.** They should say exactly what you want to achieve.

- **Measurable.** You should know when you have achieved them and about how long it will take.

- **Realistic.** The goals you set should fit your lifestyle and your budget.

- **Important to you.** Set goals that you will be excited to achieve.

Your care team is there to help you manage your diabetes. Take charge of your diabetes! Start by listing your goals on the following pages.

My goals for blood glucose

Mark the times you should check your blood glucose. Then write down your blood glucose goals.

❑ Before meals: _____

❑ After meals: _____

❑ Bedtime: _____

My A1c should be: _____

I plan to reach these goals by:

My goal for my blood pressure is _____

I plan to reduce my blood pressure by:

My goals for my cholesterol and triglycerides

Total cholesterol _____   LDL _____

Triglycerides _____   HDL _____

I plan to reduce my cholesterol by:

My goals for preventing infections and protecting my teeth, eyes, kidneys and feet

- ❏ I will visit my dentist _____ time(s) a year.

- ❏ I will visit my eye doctor _____ time(s) a year.

- ❏ I will have my urine tested for protein _____ time(s) a year.

- ❏ I will check my feet _____ time(s) a day.

- ❏ I will take my shoes and socks off at every doctor appointment and remind my doctor to examine my feet.

- ❏ If I smoke, here is how I plan to quit:

- ❏ If my doctor has prescribed a daily aspirin for me, I will take it as prescribed.

- ❏ I will have a flu shot every year.

My activity goals

1. Activities that are safe and practical for me to do regularly:

2. Types of activities I enjoy:

3. Where I can do my exercises:

4. The times of day that are best for me to exercise:

5. The times of day when I can exercise 30 minutes or longer:

6. The days of the week when I have time to exercise:

7. What I will carry to prevent hypoglycemia (low blood glucose),
    if this is a risk for me:

8. How I will track my progress as I exercise:

My goals for healthy eating

1. What is good about the way I eat?

2. What is not good about the way I eat?

3. What is one thing I can do right now to improve the way I eat?

4. What can I do long-term to improve the way I eat?

5. How will I begin to make these changes?

Food Records

Many people find it helpful to record the foods they eat, what times they eat and how many carbohydrates they eat. If you also keep track of your blood glucose levels, diabetes medicine and physical activity, you will get a better picture of how food, activity and medicine affect your blood glucose. Ask your dietitian for a food record, or make your own.

My food plan

Together, you and your dietitian to will create a meal plan that's right for you. Write down the number of food servings you're allowed at each meal and snack. (Food servings are sometimes called food "choices" or "units.") Then use the sample serving sizes on pages 170 and 171 to decide what you will eat.

Your dietitian may ask you to eat a certain number of servings of carbohydrates ("carbs"), meat and fat at each meal. For example, if you are allowed 3 carbs, 1 meat and 1 fat for breakfast, you could have:

> 1 cup cooked cereal (2 carb servings)
>
> 1 slice whole grain toast with 1 teaspoon soft tub margarine (1 carb and 1 fat serving)
>
> 3 ounces Canadian bacon (1 meat serving)
>
> Sugar-free jelly ("free" food)

"Free" foods are non-starchy vegetables (like celery, lettuce, cucumbers, peppers, onions) and condiments (such as ketchup, mustard and sugar-free jelly).

nI = 24 Need approx. 2200-2400 Calories
for healing after surgery
16-18 carb servings per day
Exercise per cardiac Rehab.

My food plan (continued)

Breakfast

- Carbohydrates (starches, fruits, grains): _____ 4-5 servings
- Meats and meat substitutes: _____ 0 -1 ounces
- Fats: _____ 2
- Free foods: _____
- Milk _ 1% = 1 carb

Snack

Carbohydrates (starches, fruits, grains): _____ ~~4-5~~

Meats and meat substitutes: _____

Fats: _____

Free foods: _____

Lunch

Carbohydrates (starches, fruits, grains): _____ 4-5 servings

Meats and meat substitutes: _____ 4 ounces

Fats: _____ 2

Free foods: _____

Snack

Carbohydrates (starches, fruits, grains): _____ 0-1

Meats and meat substitutes: _____

Fats: _____

Free foods: _____

Dinner

Carbohydrates (starches, fruits, grains): _____ 4-5

Meats and meat substitutes: _____ 4

Fats: _____ 2

Free foods: _____

Snack

Carbohydrates (starches, fruits, grains): _____ 1

Meats and meat substitutes: _____ 1

Fats: _____

Free foods: _____

Carbs

Sample serving sizes

To measure one carb, meat or fat serving, use the list below.

One carb serving is the same as:

One starch:

1 bread slice or roll (whole wheat, rye, pumpernickel or white)

1 6-inch tortilla

1 waffle or pancake

½ English muffin, pita, hot dog bun or hamburger bun

¼ large bagel

¾ cup dry cereal

½ cup cooked cereal

1 cup soup

4 to 6 crackers

⅓ cup cooked rice or pasta

½ cup cooked corn, sweet potato, white potato or legumes (dried beans, peas or lentils)

1 cup winter squash

¾ cup pretzels, potato chips or tortilla chips

3 cups popped popcorn

One fruit:

1 small fresh fruit

½ cup canned fruit

¼ cup dried fruit

17 small grapes

½ cup fruit juice

1 cup melon

1 cup berries

2 tablespoons raisins

One milk:

1 cup fat-free or low-fat milk

⅔ cup fat-free yogurt (plain or flavored)

1 cup soymilk

One "other":

2-inch square of cake or brownie

2 small cookies

½ cup ice cream or frozen yogurt

¼ cup sherbet or sorbet

1 tablespoon syrup, jam, jelly, sugar or honey

1 carb = 1 starch or 1 fruit or 1 milk = 15 grams carbohydrate

One serving of meat or meat substitute is the same as:

3 ounces cooked chicken, turkey, fish, beef, pork, wild game
3 ounces low-fat cheese
1 cup cottage cheese
1 cup tuna
1 cup tofu
3 tablespoons peanut butter
3 eggs

One serving of fat is the same as:

1 teaspoon margarine, butter, oil, mayonnaise
1 tablespoon cream cheese, salad dressing, reduced-fat margarine, reduced-fat mayonnaise
1 tablespoon nuts or seeds
2 tablespoons sour cream, low-fat cream cheese

One serving of free foods is the same as:

1 cup raw vegetables such as celery, green beans, tomatoes, salad greens, zucchini
½ cup cooked vegetables
½ cup tomato or other vegetable juice
Any amount of sugar-free, fat-free condiment (such as ketchup, mustard, sugar-free jelly)

My weight management goals

1.

2.

3.

My stress management goals

1.

2.

3

My support system

Fill in the following sections. Be as specific as you can. As you write your ideas, think about all the things you must do to manage your diabetes—eating healthy, staying physically active, checking your blood glucose, taking medicines and coping emotionally.

1. My family and friends make it easier to manage diabetes by:

2. My family and friends make it harder to manage diabetes by:

3. I wish they would help me manage diabetes by:

4. My health care team can help me manage diabetes by:

My checklist for doctor's visits

Test	How often	Goal	Result		
			Date:	Date:	Date:
A1c	Every 3 to 6 months	Under 7%			
Blood pressure	Every visit	Under 130/80			
Triglycerides	Every year	Under 150			
Cholesterol	Every year	Under 200			
LDL (bad cholesterol)	Every year	Under 100 (under 70 if you have heart disease)			
HDL (good cholesterol)	Every year	Men: over 40 Women: over 50			
Weight	Every visit	_____ lbs			
Feet (mono-filament)	Every visit	Sensation in feet. No cuts or sores.			
Urine (micro-albumin)	Every year	Under 30			
Eyes	Every year	No changes in retina			

My medications and supplements

Name	Dose	When to take it	What it does

Web Resources

General health and diabetes resources

American Diabetes Association: www.diabetes.org

International Diabetes Federation: www.idf.org

American Heart Association: www.americanheart.org

Food and Drug Administration: www.fda.gov

National Diabetes Education Program:
www.ndep.nih.gov/diabetes/prev/prevention.htm

Web MD: www.webmd.com

Exercise

American College of Sports Medicine: www.acsm.org/sportsmed

Cooper Institute: www.cooperinst.org

Nutrition

American Dietetic Association: www.eatright.org

Tufts Nutrition Navigator: navigator.tufts.edu

Food and Fitness Journaling: www.fitday.com

USDA nutrient database:
www.nal.usda.gov/fnic/cgi-bin/nut_search.pl

Calorie King (nutrient database):
www.calorieking.com

My Pyramid (food guide pyramid):
www.mypyramid.gov

Health fraud

Quackwatch: www.quackwatch.com

Glossary

A1c (also called HbA1c, or glycosylated hemoglobin). A blood test done by your care provider. It shows how you have controlled your blood glucose over the past three months.

Aerobic activity. Physical activity (such as walking, swimming and cycling) that increases your heart rate for a time. Aerobic activities require repeated motion of major muscle groups like those in the arms and legs.

Alpha-glucosidase inhibitors. Oral medicines that slow the absorption of carbohydrate. This helps keep your blood glucose from rising too high after meals. For type 2 diabetes.

Biguanides. Oral medicines that keep the liver from releasing too much glucose. They may help reduce insulin resistance. For type 2 diabetes.

Blood glucose level (also called blood sugar level). The amount of glucose in your bloodstream. See *glucose, fasting blood glucose level* and *non-fasting blood glucose level.*

Blood glucose record. Daily record of your blood glucose results and the time and dose of medicines taken. Includes anything that may affect your blood glucose, such as stress, illness or change in your activity level.

Blood glucose meter. A small machine used to measure the level of glucose in the blood.

Carbohydrate. The main source of energy for the body. Foods that contain carbohydrate are grains, fruits, milk, desserts, starchy vegetables (such as corn or potatoes) and legumes (dried beans, peas and lentils).

Carbohydrate counting. A tool to guide how you plan your meals and take your diabetes medicine.

Certified diabetes educator. Health care professionals (nurses, dietitians, pharmacists, doctors, exercise physiologists, podiatrists and social workers) who specialize in the care and education of people with diabetes.

Circulation. Blood flow in the body.

Combination medicine. Oral medicine that contains two types of medicine in one pill. For type 2 diabetes.

Cholesterol. Wax-like substance found in animal products.

Diabetes. Disease that results when the pancreas cannot produce enough insulin or the body has trouble using insulin (insulin resistance). Marked by high blood glucose levels in the bloodstream.

Diabetes treatment plan. The tools that you and your diabetes care team design to manage your diabetes. These basic skills for daily living include nutrition, physical activity, medicine and testing your blood glucose.

Diabetic nephropathy. Kidney damage resulting from long-term high blood glucose. Untreated, this can lead to kidney failure.

Diabetic retinopathy. Vision problems that result when the tiny blood vessels of the retina leak or break. May lead to blindness. Caused by long-term high blood glucose.

Duration. The period of time in which insulin works to lower blood glucose.

Endocrinologist. A doctor who specializes in how hormones, including insulin, affect the body.

Exchange lists. A tool to guide your meal planning. It defines portion sizes and groups together foods with similar nutritional values (for carbohydrate, protein, fat and calories). This allows foods to be "traded" within a group.

Fasting blood glucose level. Amount of glucose in your bloodstream after you go without any calories for at least eight hours.

Fat. A nutrient vital for your body to work properly.

Food diary. A tool to keep track of the food you eat throughout the day.

Food pyramid (also called My Pyramid). A tool to help you make healthier food choices. Divides foods into six food groups.

Food label. See *nutrition facts label.*

Gestational diabetes. Diabetes that occurs during pregnancy, often in the last trimester.

Glucose. A type of sugar that the body uses for energy with the help of insulin. Most of the food we eat changes to glucose.

Glycemic index. A way of ranking foods based on how they affect your blood glucose levels.

Goals. See *long-term goals.*

High blood pressure (hypertension). A higher than normal force of blood pressing against the walls of your arteries.

Hyperglycemia. High blood glucose or too much glucose in the bloodstream.

Hyperglycemic. Being in a state of hyperglycemia.

Hypoglycemia. Low blood glucose or not enough glucose in the bloodstream.

Hypoglycemic. Being in a state of hypoglycemia.

Impaired fasting glucose (also called IFG or pre-diabetes). When your blood glucose level is higher than normal, but not high enough to be diabetes. (Blood glucose level is 100 to 125 within two hours of eating.)

Impaired glucose tolerance (also called IGT or pre-diabetes). When your blood glucose level is higher than normal, but not high enough to be diabetes. (Blood glucose level of 140 to 199 within two hours of eating.)

Insulin. Hormone made by the pancreas in response to rising blood glucose levels. Insulin makes it possible for the cells of the body to take in glucose from the bloodstream. The glucose is then used for energy or stored for later use.

Insulin resistance. When the body's cells have trouble using insulin. It may be caused by being overweight, aging, high blood pressure or high cholesterol.

Intermediate-acting insulin. Injected insulin that begins to work in two to four hours, works hardest at six to twelve hours, and lasts for a total of about 10 to 18 hours.

Lancet. A tiny needle used in a lancing device. See *lancing device.*

Lancing device. A tool that makes it easier to prick your finger and collect blood for blood glucose testing.

Liver. A large organ that regulates blood glucose. It stores extra glucose and releases it back into the bloodstream when blood glucose levels are low.

Long-acting insulin. A type of injected insulin that works for about 24 hours.

Long-term complications. Health problems that result from having high blood glucose levels for a number of years. They include damage to nerves, large blood vessels and small blood vessels.

Long-term goals. A desired outcome that can be measured. These goals are often achieved through several steps or smaller goals.

Meglitinides. Oral medicines that help the body release insulin more quickly in response to food. They help keep blood glucose from rising too high after meals. For type 2 diabetes.

Microalbumin. Small amounts of proteins that, if found in your urine, can be a sign of kidney disease.

Milligrams per deciliter (mg/dl). The way your meter reads the amount of glucose in your blood (weight/volume).

Mixed dose of insulin. A combination of longer-acting and shorter-acting insulins given at the same time.

Monofilament. A thin nylon wire attached at one end to a handle. Used to check for nerve damage in your feet.

Neuropathy. Nerve damage resulting from long-term high blood glucose. Symptoms include pain, loss of feeling and muscle weakness (often in the hands, legs and feet). Nerve damage may also affect the heart, bladder, digestive system and sexual organs.

Non-fasting blood glucose level. Amount of glucose in your bloodstream when you have eaten within eight hours.

Nutrition facts label (also called food label). A label found on every pre-packaged food at the grocery store. It lists the food's basic nutrients.

Ophthalmologist. A doctor who specializes in eye care.

Optometrist. A doctor who specializes in correcting vision problems.

Pancreas. A small organ below your liver that produces insulin.

Peak. The period of time when diabetes medicines are working hardest to lower blood glucose.

Pedorthist. Footwear specialist.

Podiatrist. Foot doctor.

Pre-diabetes. When your blood glucose level is higher than normal, but not high enough to be diabetes.

Protein. A nutrient that helps make and repair muscles and organs.

Rapid-acting insulin. Injected insulin that begins to work within 15 minutes, works hardest at 30 minutes to 1½ hours, and lasts for a total of three to four hours.

Registered dietitian (RD). A health care professional specializing in nutrition.

Registered nurse (RN). A health care professional specializing in the maintenance of health.

Retinopathy. See *Diabetic retinopathy.*

Risk factors. Health concerns that put you at risk for serious health problems. They include things you can control, such as high blood pressure, high LDL cholesterol or low HDL cholesterol, high triglyceride levels, smoking, inactivity or being overweight. They also include things you cannot control, such as age, gender, family history and ethnic background.

Self-management. Taking an active role in making and using your diabetes treatment plan.

Serving. A measured amount of food. If you know how many servings you are eating, you can figure out the amount of nutrients you are getting from your food.

Sharps. Needles used for checking blood glucose (also called lancets) or for injecting insulin. Used sharps require special storage and disposal.

Sharps container. A special container used to safely store used sharps.

Short-acting insulin. Injected insulin that begins to work in 30 minutes to an hour, works hardest at two to three hours, and lasts for a total of three to six hours.

Sick day plan. A plan, written by you and your diabetes care team, to follow on days when you are sick. It tells you how often to test your blood glucose, what to eat and drink and when to call your care team.

Sulfonylureas. Oral medicines that lower blood glucose by helping the body produce more insulin. For type 2 diabetes.

Thiazolidinediones. Oral medicines that decrease insulin resistance in muscle cells, helping them use blood glucose for energy. For type 2 diabetes.

Triglycerides. Blood fats.